THE
SKIN-HEALTH
CONNECTION:
The Ultimate Guide to Support Your Skin Health from the Inside Out

Joanna Bacchus

complete information. No warranties of any kind are expressed or implied. Readers acknowledge that the author is not engaging in the rendering of legal, financial, medical or professional advice. The content of this book has been derived from various sources. Please consult a licensed professional before attempting any techniques outlined in this book.

By reading this document, the reader agrees that under no circumstances is the author responsible for any losses, direct or indirect, which are incurred as a result of the use of information contained within this document, including, but not limited to, —errors, omissions, or inaccuracies.

DEDICATION

This book is for everyone who's struggled with skin problems and felt overwhelmed by all the confusing advice and instant solutions out there. It's here to help you get to grips with what really works, heal your skin, and finally enjoy having clear, healthy skin. This is all about taking good care of yourself, both inside and out. Cheers to feeling great about your skin, finding out what's actually true about taking care of it, and feeling confident in your own skin.

TABLE OF CONTENTS

Conclusion

INTRODUCTION

A Journey to Radiant Skin: My Personal Path to Healing

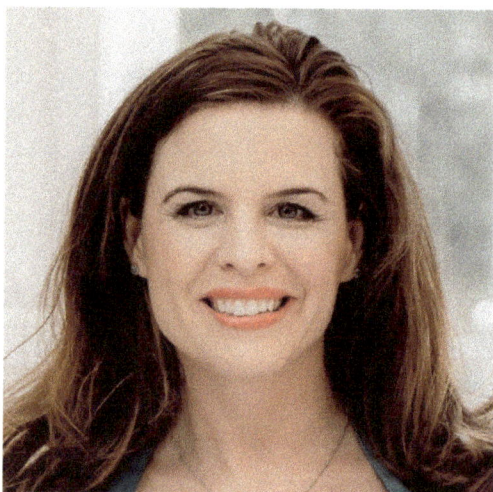

A Personal Journey to Acne-Free Skin

I started dealing with acne when I was 14 and it stuck around into my 20s. It was tough on my confidence. Every new breakout made me feel worse, thinking others were judging me just for how my skin looked. I tried everything to hide it – my hair, hats, loads of makeup. However, nothing really worked; the acne always came back. It made me feel insecure all the time.

I went through so many treatments and home remedies, looking for a quick fix, but often they just made things worse. Some left my skin dry, others just caused more breakouts. It was like taking one step forward and two steps back.

Everything changed when I met an esthetician at a beauty shop who talked about taking care of my skin in a holistic way. She mentioned diet, mental health, exercise, and specific skin treatments. It was the first time I felt hopeful. Following her advice wasn't easy; it meant changing a lot of my habits. I started eating better, working out, and treating my skin with care. I also did a lot of my own research and realized healing my skin meant looking after my whole body.

Eventually, I began to see a big difference. Not just with my acne, but additionally I felt better about myself too. It went far beyond looking good for me, I also wanted to feel good inside and out.

This whole experience taught me real beauty is

about facing and dealing with your problems, not hiding them. Now, I want to help others who are going through the same thing. This book is all about sharing what I've learned, hoping to make the journey easier for someone else. It's for anyone who's fed up with covering up their skin and is ready to find their way to clear, healthy skin like I did.

Who This Book is Not For

However, it's important to note who this book is not for. If you're seeking a quick fix, this is not the book for you. The methods and insights I share here require time to see results and involve a continuous commitment to your health. There are no overnight solutions; effective skincare is about consistent care and holistic changes.

If you are expecting instant results, you might find the journey frustrating. This book doesn't endorse one-time solutions or quick fixes which, while effective for some, can also come with serious side effects. Instead, this guide emphasizes a sustained approach to managing skin health through diet, lifestyle adjustments, and self-care practices.

Embracing this guide means you're ready to commit to a long-term journey of wellness that supports both your internal and external health. There's a detox phase, a healing phase, and a maintenance phase, each crucial to achieving and sustaining clear, glowing skin. If you're not ready to prioritize this level of care for yourself, then this might not be the right fit.

If you are ready to embrace this journey and commit to the changes needed, then let's get started on the path to a healthier, more radiant you.

A Journey of Transformation and Commitment

"Healthy Skin from Within: The Natural Path to Radiance" is all about understanding how our internal health affects our skin. Once again, this book isn't about quick fixes for skin issues. It's more about taking a deep dive into why these problems happen in the first place, often because of what's going on inside our bodies.

Your skin shows what's happening inside your body and completely fixing any issues can take a long time. We're used to quick solutions like pills or creams that don't really get to the bottom of the problem. However, this book looks at things differently, especially how our gut health plays a huge part in our skin's condition. For example, there's a lot of new research out there showing a clear connection between the health of our gut and issues like acne or even skin cancer.

This guide is for anyone who's ready to really work on their skin health in a holistic way. It's going to take some effort, learning about detoxing, healing, and keeping your skin healthy in the long run. Nevertheless, if you're up for it, this book will show you how to tackle skin problems at their core, leading to better-looking skin and a healthier life overall.

As you read through the book, be ready to see some big changes, in your skin, mind, and health. You'll be getting to know your body better and learning how to take care of it. So, if you're looking for your skin to be healthier and glow, then let's read closely my roadmap for skin health.

CHAPTER 1: NOURISHING FROM WITHIN

"Let food be thy medicine and medicine be thy food." – Hippocrates

The Diet-Skin Connection: Understanding the Impact

The idea that "You are what you eat" really shows when it comes to your skin. What you eat directly affects your skin's health, making it look either great or … not so great.

Lately, studies have been showing a strong connection between the health of your gut and different skin problems like eczema, acne, and even skin cancer. This link is called the gut-skin axis. It highlights how important a healthy gut is for good skin. Your gut microbiome, which is all the bacteria living in your stomach, has a big job in keeping this balance. If your gut bacteria is off, it can cause inflammation, and you might see the effects of this on your skin.

A Personal Story of Transformation
My aunt, who would prefer to stay unnamed,

suffered terribly from psoriasis that spread from her hands up to her elbows and across her chest. She was incredibly self-conscious, wearing long sleeves and gloves year-round to cover her skin, which would peel painfully. Finally, I encouraged her to consult my naturopath.

After some tests, they discovered she had an imbalance in her gut bacteria among other issues. They recommended a complete diet overhaul, especially eliminating wheat, cow dairy, gluten, and sugars. The detox phase for her psoriasis was extensive, lasting at least four months, much longer than typical detoxes. After four months, she began to see significant improvements. Her skin started clearing, first receding down her arms, and by six months, her chest was clear. It took a full year, however her hands healed completely eight months later and the psoriasis has never returned. She still sticks to the maintenance diet suggested by the naturopath, proving how critical diet can be to managing skin health.

Personalized Nutrition: Eating for Your Blood Type

The idea of eating based on your blood type, like what's in Dr. Peter D'Adamo's book "Eat Right for Your Blood Type," is getting popular because it helps with the gut-skin connection. The basic point is that depending on your blood type, certain foods can be good or bad for your gut health. For example, if you're a type O, eating red meat is usually fine, on the other hand if you're a type A, you might do better with vegetarian foods.

Changing what you eat to fit your blood type can also really help your skin. Even foods that are usually seen as healthy might not work well for everyone. Things like dairy, wheat, sugar, and corn syrup often cause inflammation, so cutting back on them can help. Nonetheless, everyone's different. For some, eating meat is no problem, then for others, especially those with A negative blood type, sticking to lean proteins like chicken and fish is better.

I recommend working with a holistic professional when making these changes.

Often, medical professionals might resort to prescribing steroids, which can lead to complications like topical steroid withdrawal. A holistic expert can provide guidance on natural and sustainable ways to manage your health, ensuring that the solutions you apply do not just mask symptoms, rather they work in harmony with your body's natural functions.

Lots of people have seen their skin get better after they started eating according to their blood type. This approach means avoiding foods that cause inflammation and choosing foods that help keep your gut healthy.

Balancing the Gut-Brain-Skin Axis with Diet

Besides omega-3s, focusing on the gut-brain axis is crucial for skin health. Eating fermented foods like yogurt, kefir, and sauerkraut is great for your skin because they're full of probiotics. Probiotics are good bacteria that help keep your gut healthy. Having a balanced gut can mean less inflammation in your body, which can lead to better skin. This can mean fewer breakouts and less eczema. Probiotics work by helping to keep your immune system in check, which can reduce inflammation that often shows up as skin problems (Bowe & Logan, 2011).

Eating these kinds of foods regularly can also help strengthen your skin's natural barrier. This means your skin gets better at keeping out bad stuff like germs and pollution, and it can hold onto moisture and nutrients better. For people with atopic dermatitis, a type of eczema, fermented foods can be really helpful. The probiotics in these foods help calm the immune system, making the skin less likely to flare up and get irritated (Li et al., 2021).

Don't forget about nourishing your brain with the right kinds of fats. Avocados and foods high in saturated fats, like coconut oil, play a vital role in brain health, which in turn influences your skin. Healthy fats help maintain the integrity of the nerve cells in your brain, supporting overall brain function and reducing stress levels that may impact your skin. So, by eating avocados and including some saturated fat in your diet, you're not only feeding your brain, additionally you're helping your skin heal and glow from the inside out.

Inflammation and Acne: The Omega-3 Connection

A lot of skin problems, like acne, are caused by long-term inflammation. Omega-3 fatty acids are super important for cutting down this inflammation. Adding more omega-3s to your diet can help tackle the inflammation that makes acne worse, leading to clearer skin. These fats are known for fighting inflammation, which is why they're great for acne and similar skin issues. They work by soothing your skin from the inside (Simopoulos, 2002).

Balancing Your Diet with Whole Grains

While it's important to know what to add to your diet, like omega-3 rich foods, it's equally important to consider what to reduce or balance. Whole grains are a fantastic addition to a skin-healthy diet because they are less inflammatory than refined grains and help maintain stable blood sugar levels, which is crucial for reducing skin inflammation. Including whole grains in your diet provides your body with essential nutrients while ensuring you don't exacerbate skin issues with high-glycemic, refined foods. Avoid wheat and opt for grains like quinoa, sorghum, barley, and spelt, which offer both fiber and key nutrients, supporting overall health and contributing to less inflamed, clearer skin.

The Role of Nutrition in Skin Health

Everything we eat tells our body how to behave, affecting our cells, hormones, and how much inflammation we have. This shows up in our skin. If we don't get enough of the right nutrients, our whole body feels it, including our skin. Skin without enough vitamins, minerals, and water looks dull and can get damaged or age faster.

Skin Disorders and Dietary Triggers

Eating a lot of sugar, too much dairy, wheat, and junk food is a big reason why some people's skin starts to have problems. These kinds of foods can cause inflammation, which can lead to skin issues like acne, eczema, and psoriasis. On the flip side, eating lots of fruits and veggies, which are full of antioxidants, can help fight off the bad stuff that ages our skin or damages it from the environment (Bowe & Logan, 2011).

People with psoriasis or eczema often notice their skin gets worse with certain foods. Trying out an elimination diet, where you cut out foods you think might be causing trouble, can help you figure out which foods to avoid. For instance, people with rosacea might see their skin flare up after having red wine or spicy foods. And if you have acne, you might notice it gets worse after eating dairy or foods that make your blood sugar spike (Vaughn et al., 2017).

A More Individualized Approach to Skin Health

How food affects your skin can be really different from one person to another. Some people can eat whatever they want and their skin looks great, while others find that changing what they eat can make a big difference for their skin. Because everyone is different, it's important to figure out what works for you when it comes to food and skin health.

To start eating in a way that's good for your

skin, you first need to know what foods cause problems for you and what your body needs. A good diet for healthy skin usually includes lots of fruits and veggies, lean meats, and healthy fats. These foods give you a bunch of nutrients that help keep your skin strong and fight off signs of getting older. Vitamins A, C, and E are super important for fixing and protecting your skin. Omega-3 fatty acids, which you can find in fish and flaxseeds, help keep your skin's natural oils balanced, keeping your skin moisturized and looking good (Pullar et al., 2017).

The Long-Term Outlook

Knowing that changing what you eat can really add up to make a difference in how your skin looks is key. Eating a diet full of good nutrients can help make your skin healthier and more beautiful as time goes on. On the other hand, if you keep making bad food choices, it could make your skin age faster and bring up more skin problems (Sies et al., 2004).

Superfoods for Radiant Skin: What to Eat and Why

"Glowing skin is a result of proper skincare. It means you can wear less makeup and let skin shine through." - Michael Coulombe

Getting to that glowy skin goal isn't just about the stuff you slather on. What you eat plays a huge part too. This section is all about superfoods. Yes, they're a buzzword, but they're foods crammed with important nutrients like antioxidants, vitamins, minerals, and healthy fats. These nutrients are big players in keeping your skin in top shape, repairing damage, keeping it hydrated, and protecting it from toxic pollution and UV rays.

Antioxidant-Rich Berries: Nature's Skin Elixir
Berries, like blueberries, strawberries, and raspberries, are great for your skin. They're loaded with antioxidants, especially vitamin C, which helps fight off harmful free radicals and boosts collagen. The high antioxidant content protects the skin against oxidative stress, which can cause premature aging, wrinkles, and dullness (Pullar et al., 2017). Berries also have vitamin A and fiber, which are good for overall skin health and cleaning out your system.

The colorful pigments in berries, called anthocyanins (an-thuh-sahy-uh-nin), help even out your skin tone and make it more resistant to environmental damage. Eating these berries regularly can make your skin smoother, more elastic, and more hydrated, giving you a younger and brighter look (Zafra-Stone et al., 2007).

Omega-3-Rich Fatty Fish: For Smooth Skin

Fatty fish like salmon, mackerel, and sardines are tasty and versatile in recipes, yet are also super good for your skin. These fish are packed with omega-3 fatty acids, mainly EPA and DHA, known for fighting inflammation. For your skin, omega-3s are super important because they help keep your skin's lipid barrier strong. This barrier is what keeps your skin moisturized, full, and bounce-back ready (Simopoulos, 2002).

Omega-3s are also great at reducing the body's inflammatory responses that can lead to skin issues, so they're really helpful for anyone dealing with eczema, psoriasis, or acne. They even protect your skin from sun damage and may help prevent skin cancer by guarding against inflammation caused by the sun (Black & Rhodes, 2016). If you make fatty fish a regular part of your diet, you might notice smoother skin, less dryness, and fewer visible lines and wrinkles.

Nuts and Seeds: Tiny Titans of Nutrition

Nuts and seeds are packed with nutrients that's great for your skin. Almonds, walnuts, flaxseeds, and chia seeds are full of healthy fats, like omega-3 and omega-6, and vitamin E. Vitamin E is a superhero antioxidant that fights off damage from free radicals, pollution, and the sun's rays (Cosgrove et al., 2007).

Eating these regularly helps keep your skin's protective barrier strong, making your skin look smoother and more hydrated. Plus, nuts and seeds have minerals like selenium, zinc, and protein, which are all skin heroes. Selenium, found in Brazil nuts, helps protect your skin from the sun and keeps it supple (Thomson et al, 2008). Zinc, which you can get from pumpkin seeds, helps your skin heal, keeps oil glands working right, and can help calm acne.

Leafy Greens: The Fountain of Youth

Eating leafy greens like spinach, kale, and Swiss chard is not only good for your overall diet but also does wonders for your skin. These veggies pack a punch with vitamins A, C, E, and K. Vitamin A keeps your skin strong and prevents it from getting dry and flaky. Vitamin C is all about boosting collagen to keep your skin firm and smooth. Vitamin E protects your skin by fighting off damage from bad stuff in the environment and helps keep it moisturized. Vitamin K helps fade dark spots, scars, and can reduce under-eye circles (Sies & Stahl, 2004).

On top of that, leafy greens are full of lutein and beta-carotene, two antioxidants that lock in moisture and elasticity, giving you healthier, glowing skin. They're also a great source of folate, which plays a role in DNA repair and might even help prevent skin cancer (Pieroth, 2018). Plus, these greens are mostly water, which helps keep your skin hydrated and looking fresh.

Brightly Colored Vegetables: A Spectrum of Skin Benefits

Eating colorful veggies like sweet potatoes, carrots, and bell peppers uses the colors of the rainbow to improve your skin health. These vegetables are packed with beta-carotene, which helps protect your skin from the sun's harmful UV rays, slowing down signs of aging and skin damage. Once we eat them, our body turns beta-carotene into vitamin A, which is super important for keeping skin cells healthy and making our skin look better overall (Stahl & Sies, 2012).

Besides, these vegetables are loaded with antioxidants that fight off free radicals, helping to reduce signs of aging. Bell peppers are especially good because they have a lot of vitamin C, which is essential for making collagen. This makes your skin firmer and younger-looking. Eating these bright veggies regularly can also help keep your skin hydrated and prevent it from getting dry, so your skin stays smooth and healthy. What's not to love?

Healthy Fats from Avocados: For a Radiant Glow

Avocados are packed with juicy nutrients that are great for your skin. They're full of monounsaturated fats, which help keep your skin moist and soft. These good fats also make it easier for your body to soak up other important vitamins for your skin. Avocados have plenty of vitamins E and C. Vitamin E is a strong antioxidant that fights off skin damage, and vitamin C is needed to make collagen, which keeps your skin firm and smooth (Pappas, 2009).

They also have carotenoids like lutein and zeaxanthin, which protect your skin and improve its look and color by fighting off more damage. Plus, the oleic acid in avocados can help heal wounds faster and cut down on redness and swelling, which is especially good if you have sensitive or acne-prone skin (de Oliveira et al., 2013). So, avocados are not just tasty but also a smart choice for keeping your skin looking good.

Green Tea: An Age-Old Skin Treatment

Green tea is packed with polyphenols, like catechins, which keep your skin healthy. These polyphenols are really good at fighting off inflammation and acting as antioxidants, making green tea a solid choice for dealing with skin issues. It can help calm down redness, keep your skin moist, and protect it from aging too quickly because of sun damage (Chiu et al., 2005).

The antioxidants in green tea, especially one called epigallocatechin gallate (EGCG), are great at guarding your skin against UV rays, cutting down your risk of skin cancer, and easing the effects of getting older due to the sun. Plus, green tea's ability to reduce inflammation can make acne less severe and calm down conditions like rosacea and psoriasis. Using green tea on your skin can also help make it more elastic and reduce oiliness and sebum production (Katiyar & Elmets, 2001).

Aloe Vera Juice: Soothing the Gut Lining

Aloe Vera is famous for helping skin, but it's also really good for your stomach. Drinking Aloe Vera juice, which comes from the plant's leaves, is packed with enzymes, vitamins, and minerals that are great for your gut health and help with digestion. It has properties that reduce inflammation and can act as a mild laxative, making it a top choice for calming down your gut lining. When you drink Aloe Vera juice, it can help fix up the walls of your intestines, lower inflammation, and make it easier for your body to soak up nutrients. This is good news for your skin, too.

Research backs up Aloe Vera's benefits for gut issues. Studies show that Aloe Vera juice can help lessen the symptoms of Irritable Bowel Syndrome (IBS), like bloating and discomfort, helping to make your gut healthier (Khedmat et al., 2013).

L-Glutamine: Strengthening Gut Integrity

L-Glutamine is an amino acid that's really important for keeping your gut healthy. It helps fix and keep up the lining of your intestines, stopping bad stuff from getting into your body, which can happen with leaky gut. L-Glutamine helps repair your gut walls and also helps the good bacteria in your gut flourish.

There's research out there that backs up how good L-Glutamine is for your gut. It's been shown that taking L-Glutamine supplements can really help make the lining of your gut stronger, which is super helpful for people dealing with leaky gut syndrome (Rao & Samak, 2022).

The Long-Term Benefits

Adding superfoods to your diet is really about taking care of your health for the long run. Eating foods that are packed with nutrients can make your skin look better and help it heal and refresh itself. If you keep up with a diet full of superfoods, you'll see your skin becoming healthier and more resilient over time.

Getting to that point where your skin just naturally glows and feels great means you get to enjoy tasty and diverse food which is also super healthy. When you make sure to eat lots of different superfoods, you're giving your skin what it needs to fight off aging, protect itself from things like pollution, and keep its natural shine. Just remember, getting glowing skin is about making sure you're eating well to take care of it from the inside out.

Balancing Hormones Naturally: Foods and Strategies

"The food you eat can be either the safest and most powerful form of medicine or the slowest form of poison." - Ann Wigmore

Hormones are like the body's messengers, controlling things like growth, energy, and how our body works during puberty, pregnancy, and menopause. They even affect our skin, changing its moisture, texture, and color. The skin can show what's going on with hormones inside our body.

Many women report an increase in skin oiliness and the potential for acne outbreaks before menstruation, while estrogen levels decline and androgen levels remain steady (Archer, 2004). . During pregnancy, hormone increases give some women that pregnancy glow, additionally it can also cause darker patches on the skin, known as melasma (Kumari et al., 2015). When women go through menopause, lower estrogen levels can dry out the skin and make wrinkles more noticeable (Shuster et al., 1975). Conditions like PCOS, with higher androgen levels, frequently result in acne, hirsutism, and greasy skin (Zaenglein et al., 2016).

Understanding how hormones affect your skin gives you insight into your overall hormonal health. During certain phases of your cycle, having foods like chia and flax seeds, which have phytoestrogens, and focusing on a diet rich in antioxidants and healthy fats can help balance your hormones and keep your skin looking good. Taking care of the link between hormones and skin through a healthy diet and lifestyle makes your skin better and also improves your overall health.

Eating to Support Your Skin During Your Menstrual Cycle

Understanding the impact of hormones on your skin can offer insights into your overall hormonal health. During various phases of your menstrual cycle, adjusting your diet to include specific foods can help balance your hormones and maintain healthy skin. Integrating foods like chia and flax seeds, which contain phytoestrogens, and focusing on a diet rich in antioxidants and healthy fats can optimize hormone levels and enhance your skin's appearance. A diet that supports hormonal balance not only improves your skin but also boosts your overall health.

Menstrual Phase (Days 1-5):

Focus on incorporating leafy greens, berries, fatty fish, lean meats, whole grains, avocados, nuts, seeds, chia seeds, and goji berries. These foods are packed with vitamins and antioxidants which aid in detoxification and reduce inflammation. Omega-3 fatty acids from fatty fish help in hormone production and further reduce inflammation, while chia seeds and goji berries add antioxidants and fiber to support digestion and overall health.

Follicular Phase (Days 6-14):

During this phase, include flax seeds, soy products, legumes, cruciferous vegetables, whole grains, nuts and seeds, berries, pomegranate, ginger, and maca root in your diet. Flax seeds and soy products are beneficial as they contain phytoestrogens that support the rising estrogen levels. Cruciferous vegetables help in estrogen metabolism, and both ginger and maca root are excellent for boosting energy and achieving hormonal balance.

Ovulatory Phase (Days 15-17):

Key foods to incorporate are cruciferous vegetables, fatty fish, lean meats, berries, leafy greens, turmeric, avocados, and chia seeds. The cruciferous vegetables and turmeric aid in liver function and detoxification. Essential fatty acids found in fatty fish and chia seeds are crucial for maintaining hormonal balance.

Luteal Phase (Days 18-28):

This phase should include a diet rich in healthy fats (avocados, nuts, seeds), high-quality protein sources (eggs, lean meats), high-fiber foods, and spices like ginger and cinnamon. Healthy fats and proteins are vital for supporting progesterone production. High-fiber foods help stabilize blood sugar levels and support digestive health, while ginger and cinnamon work to reduce inflammation and assist in blood sugar control.

Important Nutrients for Hormonal Health

Hormones play a huge role in how our bodies

function, affecting our moods, how our bodies use energy, and even how our skin looks. Eating the right nutrients is key to keeping our hormones balanced. This means that just changing what you eat or how you live won't be enough without focusing on some key nutrients that help keep our hormones working right.

Vitamin D, also known as the "sunshine vitamin," is super important for our hormones. It helps make sure we have the right levels of hormones and not having enough of it can lead to mood swings and skin problems. Vitamin D helps our bodies use calcium, yet it also makes a big difference in keeping our hormones like insulin and thyroid hormones in check (Holick, 2007).

Magnesium, a mineral that participates in over 300 enzymatic activities in the body, is essential for hormone production and regulation. It's involved in reactions in our bodies, including making hormones and keeping our blood sugar and blood pressure steady. Eating foods like nuts, whole grains, and green veggies, which have a lot of magnesium, can help keep your hormones happy (Sartori et al., 2012).

Another element that is important for skin and hormonal health is zinc. You can find it in foods like pumpkin seeds, lentils, and beef. It helps control how much oil your skin makes and is good for managing acne. Zinc also helps make and manage hormones like testosterone, which means it can impact a lot of different parts of your health, from how your skin looks to your immune system (Gupta et al., 2014).

Lastly, B vitamins and potassium are really important but don't get as much attention as they should. They help your cells work right, including making and controlling hormones. B vitamins, found in greens, avocados, and bananas, are crucial for making energy and brain chemicals. Potassium helps manage fluids in your body and sends nerve signals. Together, they help make sure your hormones and cells are working as they should, which you can see in healthy, glowing skin.

Hormone Health-Boosting Foods and Foods to Watch Out For

The food we eat is super important when it comes to balancing our hormones and getting that healthy skin glow. Adaptogenic herbs, foods full of fiber, and good fats each have their own special role in this process.

Foods loaded with fiber, such as beans, lentils, are key for a healthy gut. A good gut helps keep your hormones in check. These fiber-rich foods help your body get rid of extra hormones, like estrogen, by sticking to them in your gut so they don't get reabsorbed, rather they are passed out of your body. This helps keep your hormone levels balanced. When your gut is healthy, you have less inflammation and your body can absorb nutrients better, which is great for your skin (Kaczmarczyk et al., 2012).

Adaptogenic herbs like ashwagandha and maca have been used for a long time to help the body deal with different kinds of stress, like physical, chemical, or biological stress. These herbs work deep down at the molecular level to help keep a steady balance in parts of the body that manage hormones, such as the hypothalamus, pituitary, and adrenal glands. For instance, ashwagandha can help reduce cortisol, which is the stress hormone. Lower stress means healthier skin and less acne caused by stress (Chandrasekhar et al., 2012). Maca root is known for helping improve how the endocrine system works, supporting a better hormonal balance (Meissner et al., 2006).

Balancing your hormones involves evaluating what you should eat less of, or avoid altogether. Some foods and chemicals might seem okay in small amounts; still, they can mess with your hormones if you have too much of the bad stuff. Knowing about these can help you make smarter choices about what you eat and how you live.

Eating a lot of sugar and processed foods happens to everyone at some point, nevertheless, it can mess with your hormones in a big way. These kinds of foods make your insulin levels spike quickly. Insulin is the hormone that helps control your blood sugar. If your insulin levels are always high, your body might start ignoring it, a problem called insulin resistance. This can lead to more serious conditions like type 2 diabetes and obesity and make conditions like polycystic ovarian syndrome (PCOS) worse, since PCOS is tied to how your body handles insulin. High insulin can also make your body produce more androgens, leading to acne and other skin issues (Gruszczyńska et al., 2023).

Drinking a lot of caffeine and alcohol can also throw off your hormones. Caffeine gets your adrenal glands working overtime, pumping out cortisol, the stress hormone. A little cortisol is fine, unfortunately too much for too long can tire out your adrenals and mess up your hormones. Alcohol can mess with your liver, which helps break down and get rid of hormones. Drinking too much can stop your liver from doing its job, leading to hormone buildup and imbalance (Zakhari, 2006).

Soy products have something called isoflavones, which can act like estrogen in your body. For most people, eating soy in moderation is okay if it's not heavily processed and organic,

but if you're sensitive to hormones or eat a lot of soy, it might have estrogen-like effects. This could mess with your menstrual cycle, fertility, and other things affected by estrogen. If you're worried about hormones, it might be a good idea to talk to a doctor, especially if you already have hormonal issues
(Jefferson, 2010).

Understanding Different Types of Soy

It's important to distinguish between different types of soy products. Highly processed forms of soy, like soy lecithin, are very different from the organic, minimally processed soy found in products like tofu. Processed soy products can be inflammatory and have been linked to negative health outcomes, including potential connections to breast cancer. However, organic, less processed soy has been shown to potentially help prevent cancer. This is evident in Asian cultures where soy is a staple in the form of tofu and other traditional dishes. The key is the type of soy you consume, so always check the ingredients and opt for organic, minimally processed soy to avoid the adverse effects associated with heavily processed alternatives.

Fats and Your Skin: The Good and the Necessary

Healthy fats from nuts, seeds, and avocados are super important, more than just for staying healthy in general, yet also for making and managing hormones. These fats help your body create hormones, including the ones that control things like reproduction. Omega-3 fatty acids are especially good at reducing inflammation in your body, which can help with skin problems like acne that often get worse because of hormone issues (Simopoulos, 2002). The vitamins and minerals in these foods are also key for keeping your skin hydrated and safe from pollution.

You can find omega-3s mainly in fish like salmon and mackerel, as well as in flax seeds and walnuts. These fats are really good at fighting inflammation and play a big role in making hormones that help control this inflammation. This is especially helpful for dealing with acne, which can flare up due to changes in your hormones (Simopoulos, 2002).

Gut Health: The Foundation of Skin Vitality

Eating healthy fats is key for keeping your skin looking good and staying young. This section talks about how fats are really important for balancing hormones, keeping your skin moisturized, and protecting it from bad stuff like pollution. It's super important to know which fats are good for you and which aren't, especially if you want to keep your skin and body healthy.

Foods like nuts, seeds, and avocados are full of good fats. Additionally, fats do more than just give you energy; they're also super important for making and managing hormones in your body. These include hormones that play a big role in keeping your skin healthy, like estrogen and testosterone. The healthy fats in these foods help make sure the walls of your cells work right, letting hormones do their job properly inside your body.

Omega-3 fatty acids are famous for fighting inflammation and are found in stuff like fish (salmon, mackerel), flax seeds, and walnuts. These fats are crucial for making hormones that control inflammation and help your endocrine system work smoothly. This is really important for dealing with skin issues like acne, which can get worse because of hormone problems (Simopoulos, 2002).

The Antioxidant Power of Fat-Soluble Vitamins

Eating healthy fats helps balance your hormones and reduce inflammation. These fats are also essential for your body to absorb vitamins that are fat-soluble, like Vitamins A, D, E, and K, all of which play a big role in keeping your skin healthy. Vitamin A is key for skin repair and upkeep, while Vitamin E acts as an antioxidant, protecting your skin from damage caused by free radicals and environmental hazards like UV rays and pollution. Getting these vitamins by eating foods rich in healthy fats keeps your skin hydrated, strong, and glowing.

Managing Your Fatty Acid Consumption

While we know healthy fats are good for us, it's important to balance the different types we eat. Omega-6 fatty acids, found in many oils, are needed - however, remember, only in small amounts. Most people end up eating too much of them, which can throw off the balance with omega-3 fatty acids and lead to more inflammation. Keeping a good balance between omega-3 and omega-6 is key for healthy skin and overall well-being.

Adding more healthy fats to your diet isn't hard. Simple changes like using olive oil instead of processed vegetable oils, snacking on nuts and seeds, and eating fatty fish can really help your skin and keep your hormones in check. The trick is to keep at it and mix things up to get all kinds of good fats and nutrients.

I wish it was as easy as buying face cream, but getting great skin isn't just about the creams and treatments you use. You also need to consider what you eat. Through focusing on healthy fats, you'll see your skin start to glow from the inside out.

Staying Hydrated: The Skin Benefits of Water

"Thousands have lived without love, not one without water." - W.H. Auden

Our bodies are mostly water, about 55-60%, so

drinking enough water is crucial for keeping your skin looking good. Water is key for so many things our bodies do. It helps with digestion, keeping your blood flowing smoothly, thinking clearly, and keeping your skin healthy and strong.

Every single cell in your body needs water to work right. If you're not drinking enough, your body can't do its job well, which can lead to all sorts of issues. For example, water helps break down fats and fiber during digestion. If you keep yourself hydrated, your digestive system can more easily take in nutrients and get rid of waste (Popkin, D'Anci, & Rosenberg, 2010).

Staying hydrated is key for your blood circulation, too. Since your blood is about 90% water, it needs enough water to move smoothly and carry oxygen and nutrients to all your cells. If you're dehydrated, your blood gets thicker, which makes it harder for it to flow and can make your skin look less healthy (Jéquier & Constant, 2010).

Being hydrated is key for your brain as well.

Even being a little dehydrated can mess with your ability to concentrate, your mood, and your memory. Your brain is mostly water—73%—so to keep it working right, you need to drink enough water (Riebl & Davy, 2013).

Switching to the outside, your skin is the biggest organ you have and it protects you from germs and environmental harm. Your skin cells, like all cells, need water to work well. Without enough water, your skin can get dry, tight, and flaky. Dry skin is also more likely to wrinkle and doesn't bounce back as easily. Drinking plenty of water keeps your skin elastic and soft. Water goes to your other organs first, so you need to drink enough to make sure your skin gets its share too. Studies show that drinking more water can really help your skin, especially if you don't usually drink a lot (Palma et al., 2015).

Bridging the Gap Between Systemic and Dermatological Health

The link between your overall health and your skin health is really clear. Your skin often shows how healthy you are on the inside. When you're drinking enough water, your body can get rid of toxins better, which can help stop breakouts and other skin problems. Also, staying hydrated helps keep your skin's moisture barrier strong, protecting you from germs and infections (Palma et al., 2015).

Drinking enough water also keeps your skin's pH level balanced, which is important for healthy skin. Water helps you sweat, which cools down your skin and controls your body temperature. When you sweat, it evaporates from your skin, taking heat with it and helping maintain your body and skin's temperature and pH balance.

The Visible Benefits of Water for Skin

Studies have shown a clear link between drinking water and having healthy skin. Drinking more water can really help make your skin more supple, deeply hydrated, and can even make fine lines and wrinkles less noticeable, especially if you weren't drinking enough water before. Women should aim to drink about 2.2 liters of water a day and men about 3 liters. This is an easy change to make in your daily routine that can bring big benefits for your skin

(Meinders & Meinders, 2010).

Techniques for Staying Hydrated

Despite the obvious benefits, many people struggle to drink enough water throughout the day. This section contains helpful hints for increasing your water intake. Finding an easy and effective approach to include water into your daily routine is the key.

1. Use a Water Bottle with a Label

Purchase a water bottle with timers or volume measurements. This visual guide can act as a daily reminder and motivator to drink water. Aim to attain particular levels by certain times, such as midday, to have consumed half of your daily water target.

2. Schedule Reminders

It's easy to forget to drink water in our hectic life. Setting reminders on your phone or computer can help you remember to drink regularly. There are also various apps available to track your water consumption and remind you to drink.

3. Connect Hydration to Your Daily Activities

Making connections between hydration and daily activities might help create long-lasting habits. Drink a glass of water, for example:

- Following each bathroom break.
- Before each meal.
- When you first wake up and before you go to bed.
- Every time you check your email or Facebook.

4. Improve the Flavor

If you're not a big fan of plain water, try adding some lemon, lime, cucumber, or berries to it. Studies have found that adding fruit to water can make people drink up to 159% more water, even those who usually don't drink enough (Szlyk et al., 2021). Plus, these fruits add important electrolytes like calcium, potassium, magnesium, and sodium to your water, making it even better for keeping you hydrated.

Citrus fruits and cucumbers are especially good for adding these electrolytes to your drink, making water even more hydrating. For an extra hydration boost, you could even add a bit of sea salt, which is a good source of sodium (Ali et al., 2018). Herbal teas and flavored waters are also great ways to make drinking water more enjoyable and good for you.

5. Consume Water-Rich Foods
Incorporate water-rich fruits and vegetables into your diet. Watermelon, strawberries, cucumber, and lettuce can help you stay hydrated while also supplying critical nutrients.

6. Keep Track of Your Consumption
Tracking your daily water intake can provide insight into your hydration patterns while also motivating you to achieve your goals. Keep track of your intake in a journal or using an app.

7. Pay Attention to Your Body's Cues
Recognize dehydration symptoms such as dry mouth, tiredness, and dark urine. Drinking water as soon as you see these symptoms can help you avoid dehydration.

8. Use Water to Begin and End Your Day
Make it a practice to drink a glass of water first

thing in the morning and again before going to bed. This ensures that you stay hydrated throughout the day and night.

9. Make Use of a Filter

The water you drink really matters for your overall health and your skin. In many places, tap water might have toxins in it that's not great for your skin, like leftover medications and other chemicals. These can get into the water in different ways, like when people flush medicines down the toilet or from farm runoff (Daughton & Ternes, 1999).

Considering a Whole Home Water Filtration System

For me, using a water filter is non-negotiable. Research, including studies cited by the CDC, links high fluoride levels to neurological issues in children, and there's no conclusive evidence showing that fluoride prevents cavities more effectively in countries where it's used compared to those where it isn't. Lead, a toxic metal, can leach into water from old pipes, posing a serious health hazard (Popular Science, 2021). Along with chlorine that is also being added, these can also make skin problems worse, like causing dryness or irritation. This is why I've installed additional filters in the kitchen and also for my kids' shower, advocating for a whole home system if you can to ensure all water is treated.

Fluoride has infiltrated our water; also, it's in many processed foods and even in some coffee due to the methods used in its production. To avoid these hidden sources, I stick to whole bean coffee that I grind myself and brew with filtered water. The push for fluoride use has been challenged globally, leading to its ban in many countries due to health concerns. Considering all this, ensuring your water is free from contaminants like fluoride and lead is crucial for safeguarding your family's health and maintaining healthy skin.

Having a good water filter at home can help a lot. It can make your water taste better, which might make you want to drink more of it, and it also gets rid of bad stuff in the water. This helps your skin because your body isn't trying to deal with those harmful substances. When looking for a filter, find one that takes out a wide range of contaminants and remember to change it as needed to keep it working right.

Hydration and Skin Health: The Science

Staying hydrated is super important for keeping your skin healthy and looking good. Recent research has really highlighted how drinking enough water can affect your skin, making it more hydrated and elastic. This gives you a solid reason to focus on drinking enough water every day.

Your skin has three main layers: the outer layer (epidermis), the middle layer (dermis), and the innermost layer (hypodermis). Water is especially important for the epidermis because it acts as a barrier to protect you from the outside environment. When you drink enough water, this barrier works better and stays strong.

A study by Akdeniz et al. (2018) tells us more about how drinking water benefits your skin. It found that drinking more water can really improve how moist your skin is. When your skin is well-hydrated, it looks fuller, brighter, and wrinkles and sagging are less likely. This study shows that keeping your whole body hydrated is key to skin health, not just using moisturizers on your skin.

The Role of Water in Skin Elasticity

Skin elasticity is how well your skin can stretch and snap back into place. Losing elasticity, which happens because of getting older and environmental factors, leads to wrinkles and sagging. The research by Akdeniz et al. (2018) found that drinking more water can help your skin stay elastic. This means that skin that's well-hydrated is better at dealing with stretching and doesn't sag as much.

Being hydrated is one of the main building blocks for how skin cells are structured and work. Water makes up part of the cell's inside, helping keep its shape. When skin cells have enough water, they function better, which makes your skin look healthier and more vibrant. Water also helps with skin's repair processes and growth.

Staying hydrated affects your skin's

environment, including how much oil your skin has and the balance of bacteria living on it. Drinking enough water helps keep your skin's natural oils balanced, avoiding too much dryness or oiliness. Plus, having enough moisture supports a healthy collection of skin bacteria, protecting against infections and playing a part in how your skin's immune system works.

Exploring Hydrogenated Water

Adding hydrogen to water—creating what's known as hydrogenated water—introduces extra hydrogen molecules, not oxygen, despite some misconceptions. This type of water has been discussed for its potential antioxidant benefits, which might help in reducing oxidative stress in the body, including the skin. While the full benefits and effectiveness of hydrogenated water are still under research, it's an interesting area in hydration science that might offer new ways to support skin health.

The Importance of Using the Right Drinking Vessels

I personally choose to drink from copper cups

to avoid the downsides of microplastics often found in plastic containers. Copper vessels avoid these contaminants and also adds to the water's quality by its natural antibacterial properties, which can further benefit skin health by reducing potential pathogens from drinking water. Also, it helps that copper looks really pretty!

Chapter 1: Key Takeaways

- **Diet-Skin Connection:** What you eat really affects how your skin looks. If your diet is missing important vitamins and minerals, your skin might look dull and tired, and it can get damaged more easily or start to show signs of aging faster.
- **Inflammatory Diets and Skin Disorders:** High-sugar diets, excessive dairy consumption, and fatty, processed meals can trigger inflammatory responses, leading to skin issues like acne, eczema, and psoriasis. Antioxidants in fruits and vegetables protect against premature aging and environmental damage.
- **Individualized Approach:** Skin's response to diet varies between individuals. Identifying personal triggers

and nutritional requirements is the first step in creating a skin-healthy diet that addresses specific skin conditions and overall skin health. Consistency and perseverance in following your personalized diet plan will lead to long-term improvements in skin health.

- **Superfoods for Skin:** Foods rich in antioxidants, vitamins, and healthy fats like berries, fatty fish, nuts, and seeds combat aging signs, improve hydration, and enhance skin's natural defenses, leading to a healthier and more youthful complexion.

- **Hormonal Influence:** Hormones significantly affect skin health, with conditions like acne, eczema, and psoriasis often tied to hormonal imbalances. Balancing hormones through diet and lifestyle changes can improve skin conditions and overall skin appearance.

- **Importance of Healthy Fats:** Fats are essential for hormone production and maintaining skin's moisture. Omega-3 fatty acids, in particular, have anti-inflammatory properties that are beneficial for conditions like acne.

- **Gut-Skin Axis:** A healthy gut contributes to better skin health. Probiotics in fermented foods help regulate the immune system, reducing inflammation and improving skin conditions like eczema and acne.
- **Green Tea Benefits**: Rich in polyphenols, green tea protects the skin from UV radiation, reduces signs of aging, and has anti-inflammatory properties that are beneficial for treating acne and rosacea.
- **Hydration and Skin Health:** Adequate hydration is vital for maintaining skin moisture, elasticity, and overall health. It helps in nutrient absorption, toxin elimination, and preserving the skin's natural barrier.
- **Mindful Practices for Skin Health:** Incorporating mindfulness practices like meditation, yoga, and journaling can reduce stress, a known trigger for various skin conditions. These practices promote emotional well-being and, in turn, healthier skin.

- **My Personal Routine:** I start my day with a gratitude practice. Before I even take a sip of coffee, I listen to a guided meditation focused on gratitude and healing. This ritual sets a positive tone for my day, helping to lower cortisol levels, which benefits my skin. Starting your day with positive energy is a powerful way to support your skin health.

Chapter 2: The Vitality of Vitamins and Minerals

"Look after your body. It's the only place you can call home." Jim Rohns

In my early twenties, instead of enjoying new beginnings and college life, I faced a serious health issue. My skin started showing signs of a severe deficiency in vital vitamins and minerals.

What started as occasional breakouts turned into a constant problem. My healthy-looking skin became marked with acne and scars, which affected my self-esteem. I realized the issue was severe when doctors pointed out my diet lacked important nutrients like vitamins A and E, zinc, and iron, vital for skin health. My bad eating habits and stress were damaging my skin's ability to heal.

Feeling guilty and worried about long-term damage, I decided to make a change. I improved my diet, focusing on fruits, vegetables, lean proteins, and whole grains to get the nutrients I was missing. I also consulted a naturopath for supplements specific to my needs.

The journey to better skin was slow. It took months to see significant improvement, with any small setback causing anxiety. Despite this, I kept going, learning to listen to my body and give it the care it needed. Gradually, my skin began to improve, regaining its natural glow and the scars started to fade.

This experience taught me the importance of nutrition and self-care, especially during your teenage years. It's a cautionary tale about the effects of neglecting our health and the importance of internal care for our skin.

I learned how essential vitamins and minerals are for maintaining healthy skin. In life, you've got to understand the relationship between our diet and skin health, as our skin can be the first indicator of internal issues.

This story isn't to scare you, rather it is to highlight a journey of realization and recovery. If you're dealing with skin problems, consider checking your nutrient levels. A simple blood test could be the start of your own path to healing.

Essential Nutrients for Skin Health: A Comprehensive Guide

Let's talk about your body's largest organ - yep, you guessed it, your skin! This amazing wrapper we're all walking around in needs a smorgasbord of nutrients to stay healthy, flexible, and let's face it, glowing and looking fabulous.

Now, picture vitamins as your skin's personal superhero team. They're not just hanging around looking pretty - they're busy repairing, developing cells, and fighting off those nasty environmental villains that want to mess with your glow.

So, how do we keep this superhero team well-fed and ready for action? It's all about your daily diet, folks! Think of your plate as a colorful battlefield where fruits, veggies, lean meats, and whole grains are the reinforcements your skin craves.

Let's break it down, shall we? Vitamin A is hiding out in sweet potatoes, carrots, and spinach - sneaky little nutrients! Vitamin C? It's throwing a party in citrus fruits, strawberries, and bell peppers. And don't even get me started on vitamin E - it's living its best life in nuts, seeds, and those green leafy veggies your mom always told you to eat.

Oh, and let's not forget the sunshine vitamin - good old D! You can find this ray of nutritional goodness in fish, eggs, and even some fortified foods. It's like sunshine on a plate!

Hang on, there's more! In this chapter, we're going to dive deep into the world of skin-loving vitamins and minerals. We'll explore their secret identities (aka functions), where they like to hang out (sources), and the cold, hard science that proves they're not just all talk.

Vitamin A:

Vitamin A is like your body's superhero, swooping in to save the day for your skin and immune system. It's got these sidekicks called retinol and retinyl esters (fancy names, I know) that are crucial for keeping your skin in tip-top shape. This vitamin is your skin's personal cheerleader, constantly encouraging new cell growth and turning your skin's immune system into Fort Knox.

But wait, there's more! Vitamin A is also your skin's secret weapon against aging. It's all about out with the old cells, in with the new. And collagen production? Vitamin A cranks that up to eleven, helping to keep those pesky fine lines and wrinkles at bay.

Now, before you start popping Vitamin A pills like they're candy, pump the brakes! Too much of this good thing can backfire, leaving you with skin drier than the Sahara and a headache that'll make you reach for the Tylenol. And if you're expecting a little bundle of joy, easy does it with the Vitamin A, mama - high doses of Vitamin A can be risky for your baby.

However, Vitamin A isn't done showing off yet. It's also your eyes' best friend, helping prevent night blindness and reducing the risk of some serious eye conditions like dry eyes and age-related macular degeneration. Talk about a multi-tasker!

If you're running low on this miracle vitamin, your body will let you know. Night vision gone wonky? Skin feeling like sandpaper? Wounds healing slower than a snail's pace? And don't even get me started on how it leaves your immune system open to every germ in a five-mile radius! These are all signs you might need to up your Vitamin A game.

Now don't panic! Mother Nature's got your back. Load up on sweet potatoes and carrots - your body will thank you. Pro tip: pair 'em with some avocado or almonds for maximum vitamin absorption.

And for all you herb lovers out there, dandelion and nettle aren't just pesky weeds. They're Vitamin A's secret weapons for your eyes and skin, packed with these fancy things called carotenoids that boost collagen and fight oxidative stress. Toss in some rosehips, and you've got yourself a natural skincare cocktail that'll have you glowing and seeing clearly!

Vitamin C:

Vitamin C, or ascorbic acid, is a must-have for keeping your skin looking great and your immune system strong. It's a powerful antioxidant that helps keep your skin firm and youthful by boosting collagen production, which smooths out wrinkles and reduces signs of aging. Research by Pullar et al. (2017) and Murad & Pinnell (2000) shows that Vitamin C not only helps make collagen but also protects your skin from UV rays and pollution, keeping it from aging too fast.

Vitamin C is also a champion at fighting free radicals, those nasty chemicals that speed up aging when you're exposed to environmental stressors like UV light and pollution. Plus, it helps reduce dark spots and evens out your skin tone by inhibiting melanin production.

Vitamin C is also famously known for boosting your immune system. If you're not getting enough, you might feel tired, heal slower from wounds, or even risk getting scurvy. Keeping your Vitamin C levels up is what you need for a healthy immune system, strong hair and nails, and supple skin. To get more Vitamin C, eat lots of citrus fruits, berries, and peppers. Herbs like parsley, thyme, and cilantro are also packed with this vitamin. Supplements made from rose hips and amla can help with absorption and offer extra health benefits, like reducing the risk of stroke and breast cancer. And if you pair Vitamin C-rich foods with iron-rich ones, you'll help your body absorb plant-based iron better, which is great for your overall health.

So, keep your Vitamin C intake up by enjoying a variety of fruits, veggies, and herbs. Your skin, immune system, and overall well-being will thank you.

Vitamin D:

Vitamin D, also known as the "sunshine vitamin," is made in your skin when you get some sun and can also come from certain foods and supplements. It's super important for keeping your bones strong and your immune system in check. For your skin, Vitamin D helps with conditions like eczema, thanks to its anti-inflammatory properties and ability to repair skin cells (Uwitonze & Razzaque, 2018).

Your skin produces Vitamin D when it's exposed to UVB sunlight, which is key for overall and skin-specific immune health. It helps with skin cell growth, differentiation, and immune function, working directly where it's made and on nearby cells (Holick, 2007).

Vitamin D is also essential for your skin's health. It helps skin cells develop properly, creating a protective barrier and managing pigmentation. While it doesn't change your skin color, it supports an even skin tone and helps prevent aging and damage from UV light (Reichrath et al., 2007).

For those dealing with skin conditions like psoriasis, Vitamin D's anti-inflammatory action is especially beneficial. The active form, calcitriol, helps reduce inflammation and skin irritation by moderating the immune response and controlling skin cell growth, making it a great treatment option for psoriasis (Soleymani et al., 2015).

Vitamin D also speeds up wound healing by promoting the production of compounds needed for new skin formation and boosting your skin's defense against infections, helping wounds heal faster (Uwitonze & Razzaque, 2018).

While sunlight is a major source of Vitamin D, depending on your skin type, too much can damage your skin and increase the risk of skin cancer. It's all about finding a balance—getting enough sun but also protecting your skin with sunscreen and clothing. You can also get Vitamin D from fatty fish, fortified foods, and supplements. How much Vitamin D you get from sunlight and your diet can vary a lot from person to person.

Vitamin E:

Vitamin E is a superstar for your skin, thanks to its moisturizing properties and strong antioxidant abilities. Made up of tocopherols and tocotrienols, it helps protect your skin from environmental damage. Teaming up with Vitamin C, Vitamin E shields your skin from UV rays, keeps it hydrated, and strengthens the skin barrier. While it's not a substitute for sunscreen, Vitamin E offers extra UV protection by absorbing UV radiation, preventing sunburn, and reducing sunburn-related inflammation.

What I love most about this amazing vitamin is that it's a fat-soluble antioxidant that protects your cells from free radical damage, supports wound healing, and guards against oxidative skin damage. If you're low on Vitamin E, you'll know about it - you might experience muscle weakness, vision problems, reduced immune function, and issues like poor balance and coordination. For your skin, a lack of Vitamin E can cause dryness, irritation, and premature aging. Nobody wants that!

To keep your Vitamin E levels up, include foods like nuts, seeds, avocados, mangoes, and green leafy vegetables in your diet. Eating these with healthy fats can help your body absorb Vitamin E better. Herbs like gotu kola and milk thistle, known for their antioxidant properties, also support skin health and wound healing.

Beyond skin benefits, Vitamin E supports your immune system and may lower the risk of respiratory infections and heart disease by reducing inflammation and oxidative stress. Research on ingredients like green tea and gotu kola shows they help support skin structure and prevent aging, highlighting the wide-ranging benefits of Vitamin E.

Minerals' Importance in Skin Health
Minerals are inorganic elements that play important functions in the health and function of the skin. They help with hydration, elasticity, and environmental protection.

Zinc:
This mineral is essential for maintaining skin health and the development of new skin cells. It is anti-inflammatory and is often used to treat acne and other skin irritations (Gupta, Mahajan, Mehta, & Chauhan, 2014).

Selenium:
Selenium is essential for the health of your skin cells. Higher selenium levels have been linked to a lower incidence of skin cancer. Selenium also functions as a potent antioxidant alongside Vitamin E in the fight against free radicals (Hughes, 2012). Just two Brazil nuts a day can give you your daily dose of Selenium.

Addressing Deficiencies: Tailoring Your Diet for Skin Health

Let's talk about something many of us overlook: how nutritional deficiencies can sneak up on us and impact our skin. Last winter, I felt constantly tired, my skin was dull, and I just couldn't shake the winter blues. Turns out, I had a Vitamin D deficiency from not getting enough sunlight. This made me realize how important it is to pay attention to what our bodies need, especially for our skin's health. Next, we'll dive into various deficiencies like iron, Vitamin D, and more, and explore how tweaking our diets can make a world of difference for our skin and overall well-being.

Iron Deficiency Anemia

Iron deficiency anemia is pretty common and can really mess with your skin health. It can make you feel tired, weak, and short of breath because it lowers your hemoglobin levels. Without enough oxygen-rich blood, your energy drops, and your skin can get dry, itchy, and you might even notice some hair loss. Plus, iron deficiency can slow down wound healing and make you more prone to infections.

If you're often feeling fatigued, have pale skin, get breathless easily, or feel dizzy, it might be time to check your iron levels. To boost your iron, try eating more iron-rich foods like beans and leafy greens. Pairing these with vitamin C-rich fruits like citrus and berries can help your body absorb the iron better. Herbs like nettle and moringa are also great for giving your iron levels a boost. Iron is not just important for your blood health; it also supports your brain function and mood. Thus, keeping your iron levels in check can really make a big difference.

Vitamin B12 and other B vitamins

Vitamin B deficiency is quite common, especially if you have a restricted diet or absorption issues. It can cause skin problems like dermatitis, psoriasis, and acne. B vitamins are highly important for DNA synthesis, cell division, and protein production, all of which are essential for healthy skin. Low levels can reduce skin blood flow, leading to dryness, discoloration, and irritation. Plus, deficiencies can cause anemia, nerve damage, fatigue, heart disease, and even some cancers. We don't want that, especially when it's so preventable.

If you're feeling constantly tired, looking pale, getting breathless easily, or experiencing tingling in your hands and feet, you might be low on B vitamins. To boost your levels, try eating foods rich in vitamin B12 like chlorella, nori, and tempeh. Herbs like ashwagandha and ginseng can help boost your energy and improve B12 absorption. B vitamins are what we need for brain function and mood, with deficiencies linked to depression and anxiety. Biotin, another B vitamin, is vital for hair and nail health, while B6 helps regulate sebum production, so a lack of it can lead to acne and dry skin.

Magnesium Deficiency

Magnesium, often dubbed the "relaxing mineral," is highly important for nerve and muscle function, bone health, and energy metabolism. But did you know it's also vital for keeping your skin healthy? Magnesium helps with collagen production, antioxidant defense, and inflammation control—all essential for good skin. A lack of magnesium can mess up these processes, leading to inflammation, slower wound healing, and higher chances of stress-related skin issues like acne and eczema.

If you're experiencing fatigue, muscle cramps or twitches, irregular heartbeat, or headaches, you might be low on magnesium. To boost your levels, eat magnesium-rich foods like leafy greens, almonds, and whole grains. Foods high in prebiotic fibers, like bananas, onions, and garlic, can also improve magnesium absorption. Just be careful with high amounts of zinc or calcium supplements, as they can interfere with magnesium absorption. Herbs like valerian and passionflower can help you relax and may even enhance your magnesium absorption. Now, time to get some Zzzzs.

Calcium Deficiency

Calcium is well-known for keeping our bones and teeth strong, but it's also needed for healthy skin. A lack of calcium can lead to weak bones, muscle cramps, and skin issues. It plays a key role in skin cell differentiation and helps maintain a strong skin barrier, reducing the risk of skin damage and infections. Low calcium levels can make conditions like eczema and psoriasis worse.

If you're experiencing weak or brittle bones, muscle cramps or spasms, numbness or tingling in your hands and feet, or just feeling generally tired and weak, you might just need more calcium. To boost your calcium levels, eat calcium-rich foods like beans, lentils, nuts, seeds, and dried fruits. Herbs like horsetail and nettle can also help with calcium absorption. It's also important to get enough vitamins D and K, as they help your body absorb and use calcium properly. Keeping your calcium levels up prevents fragile bones, as well as keeping your skin healthy and resilient.

However, be careful with calcium supplements. While they can be helpful, taking them improperly can cause problems like arterial calcification or kidney stones. That's why it's best to get your calcium from food sources whenever possible.

Recent studies have shown that too much

calcium from supplements can increase the risk of heart disease and, as mentioned, kidney stones. This highlights the importance of getting most of your calcium through your diet and using supplements only when necessary and under a healthcare provider's guidance.

If you're thinking about taking supplements, talk to your healthcare provider to make sure you're using them correctly and to discuss alternatives like increasing your dietary intake or using supplements that are better absorbed by your body.

Omega-3 Fatty Acid Deficiency

Omega-3 fatty acids are amazing for brain function, heart health, and keeping your skin in top shape, thanks to their powerful anti-inflammatory properties. They help maintain your skin's natural oil barrier, which prevents moisture loss, reduces redness and irritation, and protects against sun damage and premature aging. Despite their benefits, many people don't get enough omega-3s, which can increase the risk of cognitive decline, depression, and heart disease.

If you're feeling fatigued and weak, having trouble with memory and focus, experiencing mood swings or sadness, or noticing dry skin and hair, you might be low on omega-3 fatty acids. To boost your levels, include foods like nuts and seeds in your diet. Herbs like ginkgo and bacopa can also support cognitive function and memory. Omega-3s, especially EPA and DHA, are great for brain health and can help reduce anxiety and hyperactivity. They also play a key role in reducing inflammation, which can cause dry, dull skin, brittle nails, and hair thinning. Plus, omega-3s are essential for heart health, helping to lower cholesterol and protect your cells by reducing inflammation. So, make sure you're getting enough omega-3 fatty acids to support your brain, heart, and skin health.

Zinc Deficiency

Zinc is a trace mineral that's essential for immune function, cell growth, and wound healing. It's also important for collagen formation, which is great for your skin. A lack of zinc can weaken your immune system, slow down wound healing, and lead to hair loss, loss of appetite, and even loss of taste. Low zinc levels can cause various skin problems like acne, eczema, and psoriasis.

To tackle zinc deficiency, make sure to eat zinc-rich foods like nuts, pumpkin seeds, and legumes. Pairing these with vitamin C-rich foods can help improve zinc absorption. Soaking, sprouting, or fermenting foods high in phytates, which can bind to zinc and reduce its absorption, can also be beneficial. Herbs like nettle, known for their anti-inflammatory and antioxidant properties, support healthy skin and may help ease symptoms of skin conditions. Horsetail, rich in zinc and silica, promotes healthy skin, hair, and nails and is also known for its diuretic effects, which help reduce swelling and inflammation.

Iodine Deficiency

Iodine is often forgotten, but so, so important for making thyroid hormones, which keep your metabolism and cellular functions running smoothly. If you're not getting enough iodine, it can lead to thyroid issues like hypothyroidism, which often shows up as dry, rough, and itchy skin. Plus, low iodine levels can slow down wound healing and make you more prone to skin infections because thyroid hormones play a big role in skin regeneration and integrity.

If you're feeling tired and weak, gaining weight despite trying to lose it, have dry and flaky skin, or notice swelling in your neck (known as goiter), you might be low on iodine. To keep your iodine levels up, try adding iodine-rich foods like seaweed (Nori, Kelp, and Wakame) to your diet. Foods high in selenium, like Brazil nuts, can also help because selenium aids in converting iodine to its active form. Herbs like ashwagandha and bladderwrack can support thyroid function and, in turn, improve your skin health.

Vitamin K Deficiency

Vitamin K prevents blood clotting, helps to build strong bones— but it does so much more. It also helps manage skin calcium levels to prevent tissue hardening and inflammation, which in turn boosts collagen production and reduces redness, irritation, and wrinkles. If you're low on Vitamin K, you might notice easy bruising or bleeding, heavy periods, blood in your urine or stool, and weak, brittle bones. These are all signs that your overall health—and possibly your skin health—could use some attention.

To avoid Vitamin K deficiency, load up on Vitamin K-rich foods like broccoli, Brussels sprouts, and leafy greens. Eating these with healthy fats like avocado, almonds, and olive oil can improve Vitamin K absorption. Plus, fermented foods like sauerkraut and kimchi can boost gut health, helping your body absorb more Vitamin K. Don't forget herbs like parsley and basil—they can support healthy blood clotting and benefit your skin health too.

Copper Deficiency

Copper is a key player when it comes to your immune system, energy levels, and collagen production. Not getting enough can leave you with a weaker immune system, making you more prone to infections, and can also cause fatigue, mood swings, depression, and joint pain. When it comes to your skin, a lack of copper can lead to decreased elasticity, slower wound healing, and issues like hyperpigmentation, sagging skin, and slow-healing lesions.

To make sure you're getting enough copper, add foods like shiitake mushrooms, nuts and seeds, and legumes to your diet. Pairing these with vitamin C-rich foods or supplements can help improve copper absorption. Just be careful not to overdo it with zinc, iron, and vitamin C supplements, as they can interfere with how your body absorbs copper. Herbs like nettle, which contain copper and have anti-inflammatory properties, can support healthy skin and help with conditions like eczema and psoriasis. Drinking water from copper vessels can also give you a little extra copper boost.

Silica Deficiency

Silica might not get much attention, but it's a big deal for keeping your skin healthy and youthful. It fuels collagen production, which keeps your skin firm and supple. If you're low on silica, you might notice brittle nails, dry and itchy skin, and even joint discomfort. To boost your silica levels, eat foods like chlorella, oats, cucumbers, and bananas. Herbs like horsetail and nettle are also great for increasing silica and promoting healthier hair, skin, and nails.

Besides helping with collagen, silica also protects this important protein from UV rays and pollution. A 2016 study by Araújo LA et al. shows that silica enhances skin elasticity and overall strength. Adding silica to your diet or skincare routine can make your skin more resilient and youthful-looking. If you're considering supplements, diatomaceous earth is a natural and potent source of silica that can help boost your body's silica levels.

The Importance of Regular Nutrient Level Checks

Maintaining the health and beauty of our skin goes far beyond just using the right creams and eating well—we also need to be vigilant about keeping our internal health in check. As we learned above, essential vitamins and minerals are crucial for skin health, and not getting enough of them can lead to a variety of skin issues. That's why it's so important to regularly check your nutrient levels, especially the ones that directly impact your skin, like Vitamin D and Magnesium.

Unfortunately, standard blood tests often miss key nutrients like Magnesium and Vitamin D. As someone who cares about their health, it's important to speak up when you're getting blood work done. Make sure to ask your healthcare provider for a full panel that includes a comprehensive range of vitamins and minerals to catch any deficiencies that could affect your skin health.

Try to get your nutrient levels checked at least once a year. Regular monitoring helps catch any deficiencies early, so you can address them through diet or supplements before they cause problems. Taking charge of your health in this way can make a big difference in keeping your skin looking and feeling great.

Chapter 2: Key Takeaways

- **Diet-Skin Connection**: Making a lifestyle change to include a balanced diet rich in vitamins A and E, zinc, and iron is crucial for healthy skin. Deficiencies can lead to acne, scars, and dullness.

- **Vitamin A**: Vital for skin cell development and repair, it promotes new skin cell growth and collagen production. A deficiency can lead to dry, flaky skin and hyperkeratosis.
- **Vitamin C**: A potent antioxidant, it enhances collagen synthesis and protects against photoaging. Its ability to reduce hyperpigmentation and improve skin texture makes it essential for a radiant complexion.
- **Vitamin E**: Protects the skin from free radicals and UV damage, working alongside Vitamin C. It's known for its hydrating effects and strengthening the skin barrier.
- **Vitamin D**: Produced through sun exposure, it plays a role in skin cell growth, repair, and metabolism. It has anti-inflammatory properties and is essential for maintaining healthy skin tone and texture.
- **Essential Minerals**: Minerals like zinc

and selenium are crucial for skin health. Zinc aids in new skin cell production and has anti-inflammatory properties, while selenium protects against UV-induced damage.

- **Iron Deficiency**: Can lead to pale, dull skin and is associated with anemia. Ensuring adequate iron intake is essential for oxygen-rich blood, necessary for healthy skin and overall well-being.
- **Vitamin B12**: Its deficiency can lead to various skin problems like dermatitis and acne. Adequate intake is essential for DNA synthesis and healthy skin cell production.
- **Omega-3 Fatty Acids**: Essential for reducing inflammation and maintaining the skin's natural oil barrier. A deficiency can lead to dry, dull skin and exacerbate inflammatory skin conditions.
- **Mindful Supplementation**: While vitamins and minerals are crucial for skin health, approach supplementation with caution. Excessive intake of certain vitamins, especially in supplement form, can be harmful.

Healthy Skin from Within: The Natural Path to Radiance

CHAPTER 3: EMBRACING HERBAL HEALING

"Nature itself is the best physician." -

Hippocrates

Ingestible beauty is the latest buzz in skincare, all about taking care of your skin from the inside out. This trend, also known as beauty supplements, revolves around the idea that eating the right things can seriously improve your skin's appearance. It champions the belief that real beauty starts with a healthy inside, so people are now taking special nutrients and herbs to help their skin glow. It's like feeding your skin the good stuff it needs to look its best.

Diving deeper into this concept, it's clear that what we eat has a huge impact on how our skin looks. We'll break down beauty supplements and how they fit into a complete skincare routine. Remember, getting beautiful skin isn't just about slathering on lotions and potions—it means nourishing your body with the right stuff. This fresh approach to beauty makes every meal a step toward glowing skin.

As we move forward, we'll also appreciate the power of herbs. Used for centuries to boost health and well-being, herbs offer significant benefits for your skin too. They work as powerful detoxifiers and natural healers, showcasing their unique qualities and the science behind their effectiveness. So, let's explore how incorporating these natural wonders into your diet can help you achieve radiant, healthy skin.

Hydrolyzed Collagen: The Building Block of Youthful Skin

One of the stars of the ingestible beauty world is hydrolyzed collagen. This type of collagen is easy for your body to absorb and is the pinnacle for keeping your skin firm and youthful. As we age, our bodies produce less collagen, so adding hydrolyzed collagen to your diet can help reduce wrinkles and keep your skin looking plump and smooth. This mighty supplement will give your skin a boost from the inside out.

Coenzyme Q10: Fueling Cellular Renewal

Another important ingredient is Coenzyme Q10,

or CoQ10. This powerful antioxidant helps your cells produce energy, including the cells in your skin. Taking CoQ10 can boost your skin's collagen production and protect it from damage that makes it age faster. It's a must-have for keeping your skin looking young and vibrant.

Vitex (Chasteberry): Balancing Beauty

Ever heard of Vitex? Also known as Chasteberry, this little herb is a superhero for your hormones. It keeps things balanced, especially when it comes to those pesky hormonal breakouts. Vitex works its magic on your pituitary gland, helping to keep your progesterone and estrogen levels in check. The result? Clearer skin and a more youthful glow.

Maca Root: The Route to Stress-Free Skin

Now, let's talk about Maca Root. This superfood from the Andes is packed with good stuff - vitamins, minerals, you name it. Maca helps your body deal with stress, which is huge for your skin. Less stress means fewer breakouts and slower aging - win-win! You're giving your skin a mini-vacation. Plus, Maca helps balance your hormones, which can lead to clearer, more radiant skin. It's feeding your skin from the inside out, helping you rock that natural, healthy glow.

Detoxifying Herbs: The Foundation of Clear Skin

Starting your journey to clear and radiant skin begins with an important first step: internal cleansing and detoxification. This is key to rejuvenating your skin, and certain herbs are especially good at this. Up next, we'll explore how to detox with these herbs and provide a practical guide for incorporating them into your daily routine.

Detoxification is essential for maintaining healthy skin because it helps purify the blood, supports liver function, and eliminates toxins from the body. These benefits are crucial, especially for tackling persistent skin issues like acne, as they address the underlying causes rather than just treating the symptoms. So, let's dive into how these powerful herbs can help you achieve a glowing, healthy complexion from the inside out.

Key Detoxifying Herbs

- **Milk Thistle:** This herb is a liver supporter. It's packed with silymarin, a compound that bolsters liver health—key for clearing toxins from the blood, which in turn enhances skin clarity.
- **Dandelion**: More than just a yard weed, dandelion is fantastic for detox. It boosts liver and kidney function, helping flush out toxins. Its diuretic properties also help remove impurities, which can improve your skin's health.
- **Burdock Root:** Traditionally used for blood purification, Burdock Root aids in toxin removal through its diuretic and digestive properties, improving conditions like acne that are caused by toxic buildup.
- **Chlorophyll**: Known as nature's deodorant, Chlorophyll cleanses from the inside by binding to toxins and removing them, which can lead to a clearer complexion.
- **Nettle Leaf**: A strong detoxifier, Nettle Leaf helps purify the blood and eliminate toxins, enhancing overall skin health.

Incorporating Detoxifying Herbs into Your Routine

Preparing Herbal Teas:

- **Choose Your Herbs:** Pick from Milk Thistle, Dandelion, Burdock Root, Chlorophyll, Nettle Leaf, or mix them up.
- **Boil Water:** Add about one teaspoon of the chosen herb(s) to a cup of hot water.
- **Steep:** Let it sit for 10-15 minutes to extract the herbs' beneficial properties.
- **Strain and Enjoy:** Remove the herbs and enjoy your tea. If it's too bitter, sweeten it with a bit of honey or stevia.

Drinking 1-2 cups of these herbal teas daily can be very effective. Consistency is key for them to work their detox magic.

Enhancing Flavor:

Add hibiscus flowers to your blend for a vitamin C boost and to enhance the flavor, reducing the bitterness of the detox herbs. If you prefer a simpler option, herbal extracts in liquid form are a convenient alternative. Just add the recommended drops to your water or tea and follow the label for dosage.

Healing Herbs: Nature's Skin Care Allies

After detoxifying, the next step is healing and nurturing your skin. This section dives into various herbs known for their healing properties, offering benefits like anti-inflammatory, antibacterial, and soothing effects. We'll help you choose the right herbs for your specific skin needs, whether you want to calm inflammation or promote skin regeneration.

In this part, we're blending old-school wisdom with the latest research to show you how to use these herbs every day. Whether you're making teas, applying them to your skin, or taking supplements, these herbs are all about helping you achieve healthier, more glowing skin.

Milk Thistle

Milk Thistle is famous for its powerful ingredient, silymarin, which is great for your liver and, in turn, great for your skin. Our liver cleans our blood, and clean blood means fewer skin problems, like acne. So, if your liver is healthy, it shows in your skin looking clearer and younger. Carlos Tello, PhD, points out in his article, "25+ Things to Try to Get Rid of Acne (2021)," that Milk Thistle can really cut down on the redness and swelling from acne because it fights inflammation.

Also, silymarin is an antioxidant, which means it helps protect your skin from pollution and stress that can make you look older and irritate your skin. This double action of cleaning and protecting your skin can really make a big difference, making your skin look younger and tougher.

A study from 2019 backs up how good Milk Thistle can be for your skin. According to research by Vostálová et al. (2019), silymarin has a double whammy effect - it eradicates skin problems yet also strengthens skin against the sun's harmful UV rays, which can cause aging and even cancer. This goes to show that Milk Thistle is a must-have in your skincare routine, giving you benefits that go beyond what typical treatments offer.

Nettle

Nettle, or Urtica dioica, might just look like a regular stinging weed, but it's actually a goldmine of nutrients. It's packed with vitamins A, C, and K, and loaded with minerals that are all great for your skin health. These vitamins act as powerful antioxidants that help fight off the free radicals that speed up aging and damage your skin.

Thanks to its anti-inflammatory properties, nettle is fantastic for tackling skin issues like eczema and acne. A study by Bhusal et al. (2022) shows just how effective it can be at reducing skin inflammation and redness. It also helps regulate sebum production, which is a boon for those with oily or acne-prone skin. Through maintaining balanced sebum levels, nettle helps keep your skin clear and less prone to breakouts.

Even so, that's not all—nettle also tightens and firms your skin, which can shrink the appearance of pores and give your skin a fresher, younger look. The youthful properties of nettle were studied by Harrison et al. (2022), adding a layer of scientific backing to its traditional uses.

Ginkgo Biloba

Ginkgo Biloba, a tree that has stood the test of time, is a treasure in traditional medicine, known for its potent antioxidants. These antioxidants are vital in fighting off free radicals that can accelerate aging and wreak havoc on your skin. Through neutralizing these harmful particles, Ginkgo Biloba helps keep your skin looking young and intact.

Even better, Ginkgo Biloba also boosts blood circulation, ensuring that your skin gets all the nutrients and oxygen it needs to stay healthy and repair itself. This enhanced circulation also contributes to that healthy, vibrant glow that signals well-cared-for skin.

Research by Huang and Miller (2007) in the Aesthetic Surgery Journal highlighted Ginkgo's benefits, showing how it can increase skin hydration and reduce roughness. Additionally, a study by Kim in 2001 demonstrated Ginkgo's protective effects against UVB damage, underscoring its role in beautifying the skin yet also in strengthening its defenses against external stresses.

Turmeric

Turmeric, often called the "Golden Spice of Healing," is a superstar in Ayurvedic medicine, thanks to curcumin, its main active ingredient known for powerful anti-inflammatory and antibacterial properties. This vibrant spice goes beyond culinary uses—it's a healing powerhouse for various inflammatory skin conditions like psoriasis, acne, and eczema. Curcumin works by blocking inflammatory pathways, leading to clearer, calmer skin.

Additionally, turmeric is effective at reducing hyperpigmentation. Curcumin inhibits an enzyme involved in melanin production, which helps lighten dark spots and even out skin tone. A 2016 review by Vaughn et al. in the International Journal of Dermatology praised curcumin's broad dermatological potential. Beyond its anti-inflammatory effects, its antioxidant properties help protect the skin from premature aging caused by oxidative stress.

Curcumin's antiviral and antifungal properties also offer protection against various skin infections.

Research continues to explore how turmeric supports collagen production and enhances skin elasticity. A 2019 study by Vollono et al. added to the evidence that turmeric helps maintain the structural integrity of the skin, keeping it firm, plump, and youthful.

Chamomile

Chamomile is essential for a relaxing tea time; however, even better, it's also a skincare champion. This herb is packed with flavonoids and antioxidants, making it a strong fighter against inflammation. If your skin is irritated or inflamed, chamomile can really help soothe and calm those areas. It works by penetrating deep into the skin, tackling inflammation right at its root and speeding up the healing of minor wounds and irritations.

It's particularly great for those with sensitive skin. Chamomile provides a gentle solution where harsher treatments might just make things worse. According to Srivastava's 2010 study in Molecular Medicine Reports, chamomile deeply soothes the skin by offering anti-inflammatory benefits from within. This makes it fantastic for reducing acne, easing skin irritations, and lessening signs of aging like fine lines and wrinkles.

Plus, chamomile does far more than just calm and heal. It's loaded with antioxidants that protect your skin from environmental stresses like pollution and UV rays, which can lead to premature aging. Studies, like the one by Merfort et al. (1994), have shown that chamomile can also protect the skin from UV damage, giving it an extra layer of defense.

Chlorophyll

Chlorophyll is an amazing nutrient for achieving clear, acne-free skin. This green pigment, which gives plants their color, is an amazing detoxifier and blood purifier. When you take it in, it significantly enhances your skin health from the inside out. Chlorophyll is full of vitamins and minerals that help detox and rejuvenate your skin.

Research, including a study by Kligman et al. in the Archives of Dermatology, has highlighted chlorophyll's role in reducing inflammation and bacterial growth linked to acne. Another study in the Journal of Alternative and Complementary Medicine by Jubert, C., et al. (2009), points out how chlorophyll binds with toxins to purify your blood, which in turn helps improve your skin's clarity.

Chlorophyll is also an antioxidant hero. It fights free radicals that can damage your skin, preventing environmental damage and signs of aging. According to Ferruzzi & Blakeslee (2007) in Food and Chemical Toxicology, chlorophyll is crucial in combating oxidative stress in the skin. Adding chlorophyll to your diet is easy. You can find it in supplements, chlorophyll water, and naturally in greens like spinach, parsley, and green algae. For an easy daily boost, just add some liquid chlorophyll to your water or smoothie.

Horsetail

Horsetail, or Equisetum arvense, is an ancient

plant and also a modern skincare hero. It is especially known for its silica content, which is vital for collagen production. Collagen keeps your skin elastic, strong, and youthful. Horsetail supports collagen production, additionally it also helps maintain your skin's freshness and elasticity.

Including all that, its antioxidants protect your skin from the daily damage caused by free radicals. According to Aguayo-Morales et al.'s 2023 study, horsetail improves your skin's mechanical properties; as well, it also boosts collagen levels, making your skin firmer.

Additionally, the silica in horsetail is essential for producing hyaluronic acid, which is known for its ability to hold moisture. This means horsetail doesn't just strengthen and protect your skin—it also helps keep it hydrated and plump.

Hawthorn

Hawthorn, known for its heart benefits, is also making waves in skincare. This plant improves blood flow, which ensures that your skin cells get all the oxygen and nutrients they need to stay healthy. Better circulation means a more radiant and vibrant complexion.

Hawthorn is a powerful antioxidant. It fights oxidative stress, which contributes to skin aging, helping prevent damage that leads to fine lines, wrinkles, and loss of firmness. Liu S et al. 's 2018 study highlights how hawthorn not only prevents wrinkle formation but also enhances skin hydration.

Moreover, hawthorn's bioflavonoids protect against UV damage, a major aging factor for skin. Keser's 2014 research shows how these chemicals help maintain skin structure and resilience, reducing damage from UV exposure and keeping your skin looking young and healthy.

Schisandra:

Schisandra is well known for skin rejuvenation. It helps replace old collagen with new, which is what you need for keeping your skin looking fresh and vibrant. The 2016 study by Guo M et al. found that Schisandra boosts the activity of enzymes that help make collagen, which means it can really help improve your skin's structure and firmness. Making Schisandra a regular part of your diet can help your skin become firmer and more elastic, reducing wrinkles and giving you that glow from within.

Rosehip

Rosehip, the fruit of the rose plant, is like a secret weapon for your skin. Rich in vitamin C, it boosts collagen production, which is essential for keeping your skin supple and firm. The high levels of vitamin C also act as a potent antioxidant, protecting your skin from damage caused by free radicals and environmental stressors, which helps keep it looking young and healthy.

As well, there's more to rosehip than a good dose of vitamin C. It's also loaded with retinoids, which encourage skin cells to grow and turn over faster. These benefits, combined with vitamin C, make rosehip great for speeding up skin healing and renewal. A 2015 study by Phetcharat L et al. highlighted rosehip's anti-aging effects, showing it can reduce wrinkles, boost hydration, and improve skin elasticity.

Plus, rosehip has essential fatty acids like omega-3 and omega-6, which are key for maintaining your skin's barrier function and overall health. These fatty acids help keep your skin moisturized and prevent dryness and irritation. Recent research by Jelena et al. (2023) even looked at how these fatty acids in rosehips can repair and protect the skin barrier, further proving rosehip's superfood status for your skin.

Shilajit

Shilajit, packed with fulvic acid, humic acid, and trace minerals, is a shout-out to ancient health practices and is fantastic for modern skincare. It boosts collagen production and shields your skin from free radical damage. Clinical studies, like the one by Neltner et al. (2022), show that Shilajit actually impacts the genes that produce collagen, giving your skin structure and health a big boost. Using Shilajit means you are embracing holistic approach to health, seeing your skin as a reflection of your overall well-being.

Prunella Vulgaris

Prunella Vulgaris, commonly known as self-heal, is packed with antioxidants and has anti-inflammatory and antimicrobial properties, making it a great choice for fighting acne and promoting skin healing. It also protects against oxidative damage and UV rays, helping to keep your complexion glowing. A 2019 study by Pan J et al. showed that extracts from Prunella Vulgaris can reduce inflammation associated with acne, making it a valuable part of any skincare routine aimed at keeping your skin youthful and blemish-free.

Creating Your Herbal Regimen: Tips and Recipes

Radiant, healthy skin involves taking care of your skin from the inside out. Using herbs in your skincare and diet is an age-old practice, backed by science, that can greatly enhance your skin health. This section gives you insights, tips, and recipes to help you develop a personalized herbal regimen that leaves you feeling confident and energized.

Understanding Your Skin's Needs

Before diving into the world of herbs, you need to understand your skin's unique needs. Factors like skin type, existing conditions (e.g., acne, eczema), lifestyle, and environmental exposures influence what will work best for you. Consulting with dermatologists and nutritionists can provide a solid foundation for your personalized herbal regimen.

Different herbs have different benefits, so choosing the right ones is crucial. Here's a quick guide:

For Hydration: Aloe Vera and Rosehip are fantastic for keeping your skin moisturized and improving its elasticity, thanks to their richness in vitamins and essential fatty acids.

For Anti-Aging: Ginseng and Ginkgo Biloba are loaded with antioxidants that help fight the signs of aging by tackling free radicals.

For Acne-Prone Skin: Turmeric and

Chamomile are great choices due to their anti-inflammatory and antimicrobial properties, which are effective in managing acne.

Incorporating Herbs into Your Diet

Eating herbs can have a powerful impact on your skin health. Here are some tips and recipes:

- **Herbal Teas:** Kick off your day with a cup of green tea or chamomile tea, both of which are rich in antioxidants and soothing to both skin and body.
- **Smoothies:** Boost your morning smoothie with powdered herbs like turmeric or spirulina for an antioxidant kick.
- **Cooking:** Use herbs like rosemary, thyme, and basil in your meals. They add great flavor and also bring skin-boosting properties.

Recipe: Glowing Skin Herbal Smoothie

- 1 cup spinach (rich in vitamins A and C)
- ½ cup frozen berries (antioxidants)
- 1 small banana (vitamins and minerals)
- 1 tsp turmeric powder (anti-inflammatory)
- 1 tbsp flaxseed (Omega-3 for skin hydration)
- 1 cup almond milk (vitamin E)

Blend all ingredients until smooth. Enjoy daily for best results.

Topical Applications

Applying herbs directly to the skin can also be beneficial. Here are some ways to do so:

- **Face Masks:** Create a paste with ground oats, rosehip oil, and a few drops of lavender essential oil for a soothing, hydrating face mask.
- **Toners**: Brew a strong chamomile or green tea and use it as a toner to calm irritated skin.
- **Baths**: Add Epsom salts and a few drops of rosemary or eucalyptus oil to your bath to detoxify and soothe the skin.

Understanding Herbal Potency and Safety

While herbs are beneficial, it's important to understand their potency and possible side effects. Always start with small amounts and do a patch test for topical applications. Some herbs may interact with medications or might not be suitable during pregnancy or breastfeeding, so it's wise to consult with a healthcare professional.

As you incorporate herbs into your routine, keep up-to-date with the latest research and be open to adjusting your regimen as needed. What works for someone else might not work for you, and your skin's needs can change. Maintaining a skin diary can be helpful to track what's effective and what isn't.

Chapter 3: Key Takeaways

- **Milk Thistle:** Protects liver health, which is key for clear skin. Its active component, silymarin, has anti-inflammatory effects that significantly reduce acne-related inflammation and redness.
- **Nettle**: A nutrient powerhouse packed

with vitamins and minerals essential for skin health. Its anti-inflammatory properties calm skin conditions like eczema and acne, and it can regulate sebum production.

- **Ginkgo Biloba:** An ancient tree with potent antioxidants that protect skin from free radicals and environmental damage. It enhances blood circulation, ensuring efficient delivery of nutrients and oxygen for a healthy glow.
- **Turmeric**: Contains curcumin, known for anti-inflammatory and antibacterial properties. It relieves redness, swelling, and irritation, and can lighten hyperpigmentation for an even skin tone.
- **Chamomile**: Offers soothing and anti-inflammatory properties, making it ideal for sensitive and irritated skin. Its antioxidants protect against environmental damage and promote skin healing.
- **Aloe Vera:** Known as the ultimate skin hydrator, it's rich in vitamins and minerals that soothe, nourish, and renew the skin. Its moisturizing capabilities provide relief

from sunburn and support cellular regeneration.

- **Horsetail**: Rich in silica, it supports collagen production and protects collagen from environmental damage. It helps maintain skin's elasticity and youthfulness.
- **Hawthorn**: Enhances blood flow and offers antioxidant protection. Improved circulation ensures that skin cells receive essential nutrients, contributing to a healthy complexion.
- **Silica**: Promotes collagen synthesis and protection. Incorporating silica into your diet or skincare regime helps maintain the structural integrity of your skin, keeping it firm and youthful.
- **Prunella Vulgaris (Self-Heal)**: Rich in antioxidants and anti-inflammatory properties, it's effective against acne and promotes skin healing. It also offers protection against oxidative damage and UV radiation.

CHAPTER 4: UNDERSTANDING YOUR UNIQUE SKIN

"The best thing about having great skin is that it makes me feel beautiful inside and out." – Kate Hudson.

Identifying Conditions and Needs: A Guide to Personalized Care

Exploring different skincare options to achieve beautiful skin is both exciting and enlightening. Every treatment and product adds a new chapter to your skin's journey towards health and radiance. This journey is deeply personal and requires a clear understanding of your unique skin characteristics and needs.

First off, everyone's skin and microbiome are different. What works wonders for you, might not work for another. Skincare isn't a one-size-fits-all deal. To get to the root of any skin issues, you often need to go through a detox and healing phase to address internal imbalances. Once that's sorted, you can set up a maintenance routine tailored to your skin type and condition.

Knowing your skin type is the aim of the game. Dry skin needs deep hydration, oily skin benefits from oil-balancing products, and sensitive skin requires gentle, soothing treatments. However, don't stop there—consider internal factors like diet, hormones, stress levels, and gut health. Hormonal imbalances can cause acne, and a poor diet can make your skin dull. Addressing these internal factors is key to lasting improvements.

Pay attention to how your skin reacts to different products and environments. Track any changes or reactions to fine-tune what works best for you.

As we discussed earlier, adding adaptogenic herbs and supplements can also boost your skin health from the inside out. Herbs like ashwagandha, holy basil, and reishi can help manage stress, balance hormones, and improve overall well-being, which all positively affect your skin.

At the end of the day, figuring out your skin type

is vital. This basic trait, largely genetic, helps you make smarter choices about the products and treatments that will work best for you.

- **Normal Skin:** This type is the dream—balanced, clear, and even-toned. It's neither too oily nor too dry.
- **Oily Skin:** If your skin often looks shiny and you're prone to acne, you likely have oily skin due to high sebum production.
- **Dry Skin:** Dry skin can feel tight and rough and may flake or itch because it lacks moisture.
- **Combination Skin:** A little more complicated, combination skin means you have areas that are oily (like your T-zone – forehead, nose, and chin) and areas that are dry (typically the cheeks).
- **Sensitive Skin:** This type reacts easily to certain products or environmental factors, often resulting in redness, itching, or rashes.

Understanding your skin type helps you tailor your skincare routine to your specific needs, ensuring you pick the right products and treatments to maintain and enhance your skin's natural balance.

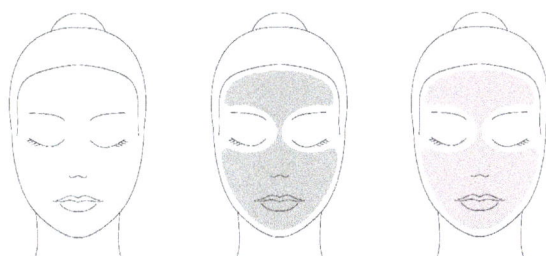

Normal   Dry   Oily

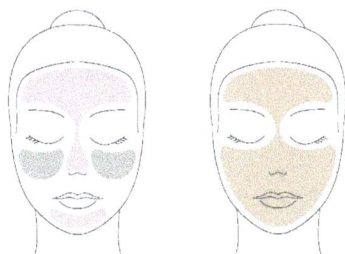

Combination   Sensitive

Once you understand your skin type, picking the

right skincare products and treatments becomes much easier. For example, if you have oily skin, gel-based moisturizers and salicylic acid treatments might work best, while dry skin benefits from richer, cream-based moisturizers and gentle, hydrating cleansers.

Dr. Leslie Baumann's book, "The Skin Type Solution," is a fantastic resource. It goes beyond the basics by classifying skin into 16 distinct types and offering tailored advice for each, helping you understand your skin's unique traits and needs.

I've got very sensitive skin, so I have to be extra careful with the products I use. Most skincare products can easily cause me to break out, and facials often leave my skin looking red. Procedures like microneedling give me the worst reactions because I'm still dealing with inflammation in my body, which shows up on my face.

The good news is that with dietary and lifestyle changes, my skin has improved significantly over the past few years. However, I still need to be incredibly cautious about what I put on my skin to avoid breakouts. One of the most valuable lessons I've learned is the importance of reading labels.

You can make a lot of natural products at home or look for skincare products outside of North America, which might be purer and free of harmful chemicals. Many skincare products here contain endocrine disruptors that can cause internal and topical issues. For any skin type, the top advice is to read your labels carefully.

Knowing your skin type is just the start. Age, hormonal balance, and environmental stress also play crucial roles. As you age, your skin tends to dry out and needs more targeted treatments for wrinkles and fine lines.

Understanding what's in your skincare products is crucial. Some ingredients might be great for some people but problematic for others. The skincare industry in North America allows many ingredients that are banned in other countries due to health risks. This has led me to seek out products from regions with stricter regulations, ensuring they are safer and more effective.

When it comes to facials and treatments, I

always inform my esthetician about my sensitive skin so they can use gentler products and techniques. Over time, I've learned which ingredients and treatments my skin can tolerate. For example, I avoid harsh exfoliants and opt for soothing, hydrating masks instead.

Understanding Your Skin Story

Achieving perfect skin isn't a one-size-fits-all solution; radiant, healthy skin means crafting a personalized routine that meets your skin's specific needs and adapts over time. Skincare is a dynamic, ongoing process that requires knowledge, attention, and sometimes professional help.

Understanding your skin type is your first step toward a glowing complexion, but don't stop there. Dive deeper into your skin's story by identifying specific issues like acne, hyperpigmentation, or signs of aging. Tailor your skincare regimen to address these concerns for more effective, personalized care.

For example, for those dealing with acne, salicylic acid can resurface even the most stubborn spots. This beta-hydroxy acid helps clear out pores by removing dead skin cells and excess oil, reducing breakouts and promoting smoother skin. If uneven skin tone or hyperpigmentation is your concern, vitamin C is excellent. This powerful antioxidant boosts collagen production and evens your skin tone, offering both brightening and anti-aging benefits.

If your skin is sensitive, choose products specifically designed to be gentle and free from common irritants like fragrances, alcohol, and certain acids. Look for soothing ingredients like aloe vera and chamomile to keep your skin calm and comfortable.

As you introduce new products into your routine, pay close attention to how your skin responds. Start with one new product at a time and monitor for any signs of irritation or breakouts. This cautious approach helps ensure you're using the best products for your skin type.

Melasma, Rosacea, and More: Addressing Common Concerns Naturally

Melasma and Hyperpigmentation

Melasma and hyperpigmentation, those annoying dark spots on your skin, are often influenced by your genes, hormones, and environment. These conditions are especially common in people with Fitzpatrick skin types III-VI, showing up as darker patches because of excess melanin, the pigment that gives your skin its color.

I personally dealt with melasma after pregnancy, and it made me feel pretty self-conscious. But I found a solution that worked wonders for me. I started using Vitamin C regularly, and it made a huge difference in clearing up those dark spots. Vitamin C is a powerful antioxidant that brightens the skin and reduces hyperpigmentation.

Over 90% of melasma cases occur in these darker skin tones, due to a mix of factors like genetics, sun exposure, hormonal changes, and sometimes even medications. When I was pregnant, I started noticing these brown spots under my eyes and on my cheeks. I couldn't figure out what was wrong until I learned that melasma is closely tied to hormones.

Treating melasma can involve light therapy and laser therapy, which are painless and effective. There are also natural topical solutions that can help. Believe it or not, potato skins can be used as a skin lightener. Potato skins contain polyphenols that can lighten your skin. You can actually put potato skins on your melasma, and many people have had success lightening acne scars, hyperpigmentation, and melasma this way. It sounds crazy, but it works!

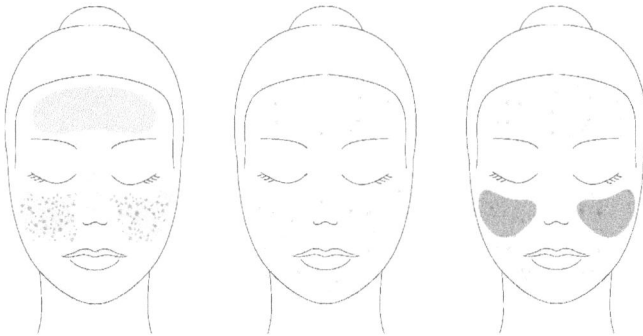

Tracing the Roots: Causes and Nutrient Links

Understanding what causes melasma and hyperpigmentation is a bit like solving a puzzle. These conditions can be triggered by hormonal changes, such as those that happen during pregnancy or from using birth control. Too much sun exposure also ramps up melanin production, leading to those telltale dark patches. Even genetics plays a role, possibly making you more prone to these issues based on your family history.

However, there's more to the story beneath the surface. Certain nutrient deficiencies also have a part to play in hyperpigmentation. Vitamins C and E, which are crucial for maintaining the skin's radiance and integrity, along with Vitamin B12 and Folate (Vitamin B9), are essential for keeping your skin tone even. These nutrients can also help you achieve brighter, more even-toned skin, and boost your health too - what a bonus.

Treatments and Nature's Remedies

There are several treatments and natural remedies that can help manage melasma and hyperpigmentation.

Topical treatments are often the first approach. Creams and serums enriched with Vitamin C, Kojic acid, and Azelaic acid work to lighten dark patches gradually, promoting a more even skin tone.

Natural Remedies:

- **Green Tea Extract:** More than just a soothing drink, green tea extract is loaded with antioxidants. It helps protect the skin from free radical damage and has properties that lighten pigmentation. Whether applied topically or enjoyed as a tea, it's a great example of nature's ability to heal.
- **Licorice Root Extract:** An ancient remedy reborn in modern skincare, licorice root is known for its skin-lightening effects and is often found in topical treatments aimed at reducing skin discoloration.
- **Gotu Kola:** This powerhouse herb is rich in triterpene saponins and phytonutrients called flavonoids, which act as

antioxidants to fight off free radical damage. Gotu Kola boosts the formation of collagen and skin tissue, which is crucial in maintaining the skin's elasticity and youthful glow. Its anti-inflammatory properties make it an excellent choice for soothing irritated skin and promoting overall skin health.To take advantage of these natural ingredients, I use a sous vide machine to blend jojoba oil with Gotu Kola and green tea leaves, creating a potent anti-wrinkle serum.

Rosacea

Rosacea is a chronic skin condition that can make your face turn all shades of red, from a light blush to a severe flush. It can come with visible blood vessels, acne-like pimples, or intense swelling. It's unpredictable, frustrating, and super sensitive to sunlight, turning every outdoor trip into a strategic mission.

Causes and Contributors of Rosacea

The exact cause of rosacea remains a mystery, however, what we *do* know suggests a complex interplay of genetic, vascular, immune, and environmental factors. If rosacea is common in your family, you might be more likely to experience it too. Your facial blood vessels may dilate more easily, leading to that flush, while your immune system might react more intensely to common triggers.

Additionally, tiny mites called Demodex, which normally live harmlessly on the skin, could be making things worse. These mites don't bother most people, but unfortunately in those with rosacea, they can cause inflammation and exacerbate flare-ups.

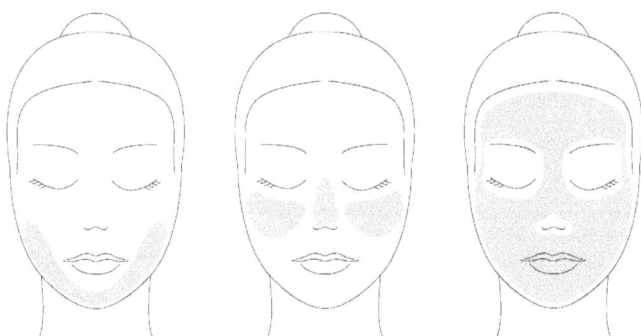

Deficiencies as Underlying Forces

Your diet might be playing a big role in your rosacea. This condition has been linked to deficiencies in essential fatty acids, vitamin D, vitamin C, zinc, and especially vitamin B2. These nutrients help reduce inflammation and protect your skin, as well as supporting

Managing rosacea is all about self-discovery and adaptability. While a dermatologist's advice is crucial, knowing the variety of treatments available can be empowering. Understanding your triggers and how to avoid them is just as important. Whether it's spicy foods that make you flush or weather extremes that trigger redness, being aware is key. Gentle skincare and careful sun protection are your daily defenses against rosacea.

Using Nature's Remedies

Nature is full of ways to help soothe your skin. Aloe Vera, known for its calming effects, can significantly reduce inflammation and redness. Green tea, loaded with antioxidants, offers anti-inflammatory benefits and can be enjoyed as a drink or applied as a cool compress to irritated skin. Chamomile, famous for its soothing properties, works well as a gentle balm for sensitive skin.

You must also take the effort to keep your digestive system healthy. Probiotics, the good bacteria in your gut, can help to manage the external effects of rosacea. When stress starts to trigger a flare-up, turning to calming practices like meditation and deep breathing can really make a difference.

Seborrheic Dermatitis

Seborrheic dermatitis can show up anywhere but is most common in areas with lots of oil glands, like the scalp, face, and chest. This condition can stir up quite a storm on your skin, leading to redness, peeling, and often unbearable itching. You might also see patches of oily or scaly skin. Managing seborrheic dermatitis involves understanding and addressing these inflammatory responses to restore peace to your skin.

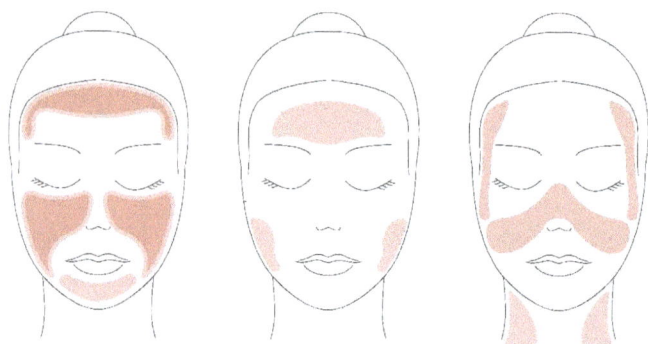

Untangling the Tangled Web: Causes and Contributors

The exact cause of Seborrheic Dermatitis isn't fully understood, and several key factors play a role. One major culprit is the Malassezia yeast, a typically harmless inhabitant of our skin that can cause inflammation when it overgrows and interacts with sebum, the skin's natural oil. This interaction can kickstart an inflammatory response, leading to irritation.

Genetics also seem to influence the likelihood of developing this condition, passing it from one generation to the next. Hormonal changes, particularly during stressful times like puberty, can trigger or worsen the condition. Environmental factors like stress or harsh, dry weather can also aggravate Seborrheic Dermatitis.

Nutritional Signposts

Nutrient deficiencies often play a big role in Seborrheic Dermatitis. Biotin (vitamin B7), known as the captain of skin health, along with Vitamin D, Zinc, and essential fatty acids, are crucial for keeping your skin balanced and healthy. Lacking these vital nutrients can make your skin more prone to issues like Seborrheic Dermatitis.

Choosing a Path: Treatment and Natural Remedies

Managing Seborrheic Dermatitis takes a comprehensive approach, combining lifestyle changes and natural remedies. Start by cleaning affected areas with gentle, fragrance-free cleansers and maintaining good hygiene to keep your skin calm.

Natural treatments can work wonders too. Apple cider vinegar helps restore your skin's natural pH balance. Tea tree oil, with its antifungal properties, can fight yeast overgrowth. Coconut oil is excellent for its moisturizing and anti-inflammatory effects, soothing irritated skin. Plus, adding probiotics to your diet can improve gut health, which in turn benefits your skin.

Including biotin-rich foods like eggs, nuts, and whole grains in your diet can support skin repair and resilience. The key to effectively treating Seborrheic Dermatitis is to focus on soothing symptoms while nourishing your skin and body to help eliminate the condition altogether.

Understanding and Navigating the Complexities of Acne

Acne is a prevalent skin condition that affects millions worldwide, often starting in adolescence and sometimes continuing into adulthood. It involves the blocking of hair follicles with oil, dead skin cells, and bacteria, leading to various types of blemishes, from blackheads to the more stubborn whiteheads.

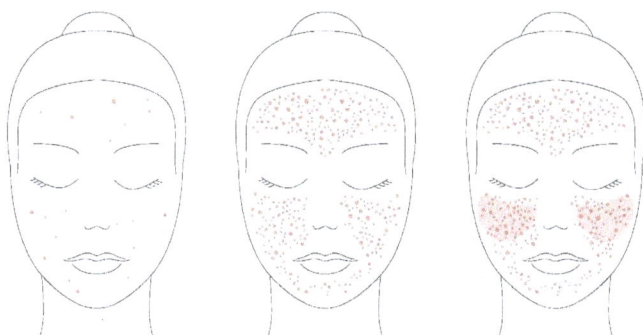

Uncovering the Root Causes of Acne

Acne is a tricky condition which is caused by a complex mix of internal and external factors. Hormones, especially androgens, can boost oil production, setting the stage for breakouts. This excess oil, combined with overactive oil glands, feeds the Propionibacterium acnes bacteria, leading to inflammation and acne. On top of that, dead skin cells often don't shed properly and mix with the sebum to clog pores, making things even worse.

My Personal Struggles with Hormonal Acne
My struggles with acne were 100% hormonal. I was literally told I had a hormonal imbalance when I was quite young. Unfortunately, I can't recall which blood tests indicated this, but I had

massive issues. The solution offered to me was to go on the pill. While it did reduce the number of breakouts, it was a Band-Aid solution. The pill caused additional issues, and I still ended up having breakouts, albeit fewer than before.

The pill didn't address the root of the problem. It wasn't until I got off the pill and started dealing with my root issues that I saw real improvement. For me, taking Vitex (chaste tree berry) and evening primrose oil, along with omega-3 fatty acids, made my hormonal acne dramatically better. These supplements helped balance my hormones, which were at the core of my acne issues.

The Role of Hormones in Acne

Hormones are inextricably linked to your gut health, brain health, and insulin resistance. They are the core piece of the puzzle, and nurturing them throughout every stage of your life is crucial. When your hormones are balanced, it will reflect on your face, dramatically improving your skin. For many women, acne is directly or indirectly linked to hormonal issues.

Incorporating Adaptogenic Herbs

Adaptogenic herbs can play a significant role in managing hormonal acne. These herbs help your body adapt to stress and maintain hormonal balance. Here are a few that have been particularly helpful:

- **Ashwagandha**: Known for its stress-reducing properties, ashwagandha can help lower cortisol levels, which in turn can reduce hormonal imbalances.
- **Rhodiola**: This herb helps improve your body's resistance to stress, supporting adrenal function and hormonal balance.
- **Maca Root**: Often used to balance hormones and enhance fertility, maca can help regulate estrogen levels and improve skin health.
- **Holy Basil:** Also known as tulsi, this herb helps balance cortisol levels and has anti-inflammatory properties that can benefit acne-prone skin.

Panax Ginseng

Panax Ginseng is a star in the world of ingestible beauty. This revered herb is famous for its strong anti-aging benefits, helping boost collagen production and fighting off free radicals. This means firmer skin and fewer signs of aging. Moreover, the perks of Ginseng go beyond skin deep—it energizes your whole body and boosts overall vitality.

Addressing Acne Holistically

In addition to hormonal balance, your diet plays a crucial role in managing acne. Foods high in sugar and refined carbs can mess with your hormones and trigger breakouts. Incorporating a balanced diet rich in fruits, vegetables, lean proteins, and healthy fats supports your overall health and can improve your skin.

Hydration is key, too. Drinking plenty of water helps flush out toxins and keeps your skin hydrated and healthy. Reducing stress through mindfulness practices like meditation, yoga, and regular exercise can also help manage hormonal fluctuations and improve your skin.

Deficiencies and Acne: A Nutritional Connection

What you eat definitely shows on your skin. Missing essential nutrients like zinc, vitamins A, E, and D, and omega-3 fatty acids can seriously affect your skin health. These nutrients help manage inflammation, control oil production, and keep your skin healthy.

Before starting any new skincare routine or diet, get your levels checked to identify any nutritional deficiencies. Common deficiencies affecting skin health include iron, vitamin D, and magnesium. Not all doctors offer robust testing, so consider working with a naturopath. This way, you're not guessing and trying different diets or products without knowing what's going on inside your body.

To get a full picture of your nutritional status, undergo comprehensive testing for levels of iron, vitamin D, magnesium, and other essential nutrients. A naturopath can help interpret these results accurately. Addressing deficiencies can significantly improve your skin health and overall well-being.

Many people struggle with persistent skin issues because they haven't addressed underlying nutritional deficiencies. Low iron levels can lead to pale skin and dark circles, making you look tired. A magnesium deficiency can result in dull, lackluster skin.

Understanding your body's needs and correcting any imbalances is the foundation of effective skincare. Instead of randomly trying diets or skincare products, make informed decisions based on your unique nutritional profile. This saves time, reduces stress, and helps achieve better, sustainable results.

In addition to working with a naturopath, focus on a balanced diet rich in fruits, vegetables, lean proteins, and healthy fats. Foods like nuts, seeds, leafy greens, and fatty fish boost your intake of skin-loving nutrients.

Treatment and Lifestyle Options
There's no magic cure for acne, but a comprehensive approach can make a big difference:

- **Gentle Cleansing:** Use a mild, non-comedogenic cleanser to remove excess oil and dirt without stripping your skin's natural oils.

- **Balanced Washing:** Overwashing can dry out your skin and lead to more oil production. Stick to cleansing no more than twice a day.
- **Hydration:** Using an oil-free moisturizer helps keep your skin hydrated and the barrier function strong, all without clogging your pores. Also, drink plenty of water throughout the day to keep your skin supple.
- **Mindful Product Selection:** Opt for "non-comedogenic" makeup and skincare products to keep pores clear.

Natural Remedies: Embracing Nature

Nature is rich in treatments for acne-prone skin:

- **Tea Tree Oil:** Its antibacterial properties target acne-causing bacteria.
- **Green Tea**: Packed with antioxidants, it helps reduce inflammation and redness.
- **Probiotics**: A healthy gut can reflect in clearer skin.
- **Honey**: Known for its anti-inflammatory and antimicrobial benefits, it's a natural

remedy for soothing acne.

A Word on Contraception and Antibiotics

While birth control pills and antibiotics are commonly prescribed for acne by non-holistic medical professionals, they don't address the root causes. True healing involves balancing hormones, ensuring proper nutrient intake, and effectively managing stress.

Psoriasis and Eczema

Psoriasis and eczema are complex challenges affecting millions. Psoriasis features red, scaly patches and is an autoimmune disorder where the immune system speeds up skin cell growth. Eczema, characterized by inflammation, itching, and irritation, often involves environmental factors that aggravate the condition. Managing these skin issues requires a nuanced approach.

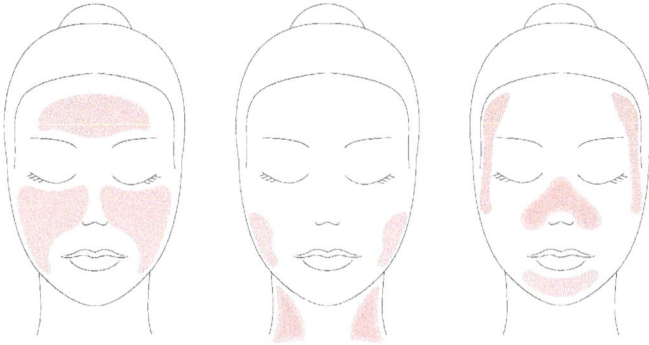

Causes and Triggers

Both psoriasis and eczema have genetic roots, so if they run in your family, you might be more prone to them. Psoriasis is an immune system error where the body mistakenly attacks healthy skin cells, leading to rapid cell growth and causing itchy, scaly patches. Eczema, on the other hand, is characterized by an overactive inflammatory response, often triggered by environmental factors and irritants.

These skin conditions are influenced by various factors. Stress, infections, certain medications, and even physical injuries can trigger psoriasis or eczema flare-ups. Eczema often involves a compromised skin barrier, which lets moisture out and allergens in, leading to inflammation and relentless itching.

The Role of Deficiencies

Missing out on certain nutrients can make psoriasis and eczema worse. Vitamins A, D, and E, along with essential fatty acids, are crucial for regulating the immune response, maintaining skin integrity, and managing inflammation. Getting enough of these nutrients can help soothe your skin troubles.

Harmonizing Treatments

Managing psoriasis and eczema requires a balanced approach, combining natural remedies and lifestyle changes to soothe and heal the skin. Regular use of moisturizers can alleviate dryness and itching—opt for natural ones like oat-based products, which are gentle and free from harsh chemicals. It's also essential to know *what* is triggering you - so make time to identify and avoid your personal triggers, and protect your skin from the sun, to prevent exacerbating symptoms.

Natural Remedies: Nature's Ensemble

Nature offers a variety of treatments, each with unique calming and healing properties:

- **Omega-3 fatty acids:** Found in fatty fish and supplements, these essential nutrients have anti-inflammatory properties that help soothe irritation.
- **Probiotics**: Enhancing gut health, probiotics can help reduce the severity of flare-ups by calming inflammatory responses.
- **Aloe vera gel**: Known for its anti-inflammatory and healing properties, aloe vera can be a soothing remedy for sensitive skin.

Premature Wrinkles and Collagen Loss

Premature wrinkles and collagen loss tell the stories of our lives—smiles, worries, and time passing. These signs often make us find ways to keep our skin youthful and elastic.

One of the best strategies is adding collagen to your routine. Collagen keeps your skin firm and elastic, but its production decreases as we age, leading to wrinkles and sagging. Collagen supplements, especially hydrolyzed collagen, can help. Hydrolyzed collagen is broken down into small, easily absorbed molecules, making it more effective. You can find it in marine (fish) or grass-fed bovine (cow) sources. The key is to ensure it's hydrolyzed for maximum absorption.

I've tried many collagen supplements and found that the market is full of products that don't work. Many have fillers and low-quality ingredients. It's essential to read labels and choose products tested for quality and purity. Avoid proprietary blends that don't disclose ingredient amounts. Opt for products with full ingredient lists and third-party testing.

Maintain a healthy lifestyle with a balanced diet rich in antioxidants, omega-3s, and other skin-loving nutrients. Stay hydrated, get enough sleep, manage stress, and exercise regularly. All these factors contribute to healthy, radiant skin that ages gracefully.

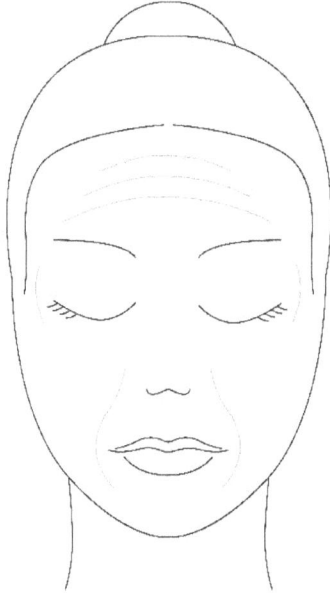

Uncovering the Root Causes of Premature Aging

Premature wrinkles and collagen loss come from both natural and environmental factors. As we age, our bodies produce less collagen and elastin, leading to less supple skin and more wrinkles. Genetics play a big role in how quickly and severely we experience these changes.

The sun is a major culprit in skin aging. UV rays damage the collagen in our skin, weakening its support structure. Pollution, toxins, and harsh weather conditions also contribute to collagen breakdown and accelerate aging.

Lifestyle choices greatly affect our skin health. Smoking, poor nutrition, excessive alcohol, chronic stress, and lack of sleep can speed up aging and leave lasting marks on our skin.

Feeding the Skin with Nutrition

To combat premature wrinkles and collagen loss, certain nutrients are essential. Vitamins C, E, and A, along with minerals like zinc and copper, are vital for collagen synthesis and overall skin health. Omega-3 fatty acids are especially important because they build healthy skin cells and reduce inflammation.

Adopting a Holistic Approach

Addressing early wrinkles and collagen loss effectively involves a holistic strategy that includes sun protection, a healthy lifestyle, and a nutrient-rich skincare routine:

- **Nourish Yourself:** Eat a balanced diet full

of fruits, vegetables, and omega-3 fatty acids to provide your skin with the nutrients it needs to thrive.

- **Stay Hydrated**: Keeping hydrated is crucial for skin elasticity. Drink plenty of water and use a quality moisturizer to keep your skin firm and hydrated.
- **Skincare Routine**: Develop a skincare routine that includes products that enhance collagen production and skin elasticity. Look for ingredients like retinol, peptides, and hyaluronic acid.
- **Antioxidants Are Your Friends**: Eat a diet rich in antioxidants to combat free radicals and environmental damage that can accelerate aging.

Taking Control of Your Skin Journey

Managing premature wrinkles and collagen loss means embracing your aging process with grace and self-care, not fighting your age or changing who you are. Today's treatments, along with natural remedies, offer many ways to support your skin's health. Your skin's journey, including fine lines and wrinkles, is unique. It reflects your life, emotions, and experiences and should be cared for and celebrated.

"Your skin is yours. Don't turn away from it when it needs you." This thought is a gentle reminder to look after your skin at every stage, embracing changes with kindness and understanding. Your skin is with you for life; treat it with the love and respect it deserves.

Chapter 4: Key Takeaways

- **Tackling Dark Spots**: Melasma and hyperpigmentation are triggered by genetics, sun exposure, hormonal shifts, and medications. Topical treatments like Vitamin C and Kojic acid can lighten dark spots.

- **Rosacea Management**: Understand your triggers and use a gentle skincare routine. Ingredients like Aloe Vera and Chamomile soothe the skin, and sunscreen prevents flare-ups.

- **Seborrheic Dermatitis**: Manage this with gentle cleansing, regular moisturizing, and natural antifungal treatments like tea tree oil.

- **Understanding Acne**: Hormonal fluctuations, increased sebum production, and bacterial growth cause acne. Treatments range from salicylic acid and tea tree oil to dietary changes.

- **Psoriasis and Eczema**: Genetics, immune responses, and environmental factors play roles. Keep skin moisturized, avoid triggers, and use natural anti-inflammatory remedies.

- **Premature Wrinkles and Collagen Loss**: Genetics, sun exposure, and lifestyle choices contribute. Eat a diet rich in antioxidants, use sunscreen, and apply collagen-boosting skincare.

- **Holistic Skin Care Approach**: Healthy skin goes beyond topical treatments. Combine a nutritious diet, hydration, sun protection, stress management, and personalized skincare for the best results.

CHAPTER 5: THE POWER OF NATURAL TOPICALS

"Nature gives you the face you have at twenty; it is up to you to merit the face you have at fifty." - Coco Chanel

Enhancing Your Skin Naturally

Nature is a generous source of solutions for achieving bright, healthy skin. Each natural remedy brings its unique benefits and healing properties to the table. Let's get right into some of nature's most effective skin care treasures:

Natural Oils for Radiant Skin

Castor Oil: Moisture and Calm for Sensitive Skin

Castor oil, from the Ricinus communis plant, is a fantastic natural remedy packed with ricinoleic acid. This thick, soothing oil is perfect for sensitive or acne-prone skin because it's anti-inflammatory and antibacterial. It locks in moisture, helping with dryness and giving you a supple, hydrated complexion. Castor oil is a classic go-to for purifying and rejuvenating your skin, showing just how powerful natural treatments can be.

Myrrh: Ancient Resin for Modern Skin Care

Myrrh, a resin from the Commiphora myrrha tree, is a historic gem in skincare. It's packed with antioxidants and anti-inflammatory benefits, making it great for soothing skin irritations and fighting signs of aging. Myrrh deeply moisturizes and can help with conditions like eczema and acne. Plus, its antiseptic properties make your skin more resistant to infections, keeping it healthy and vibrant.

Frankincense: The King of Oils

Frankincense, known as the "king of oils," comes from the resin of the Boswellia tree and has been cherished for centuries. It's not only loved for its aroma but also for its amazing health benefits. Frankincense is great for rejuvenating the skin, reducing scars and wrinkles, and promoting overall skin health.

However, not all frankincense is created equal. Genuine frankincense oil is carefully extracted to preserve its beneficial compounds, while many products on the market are diluted or mixed with synthetic ingredients, which can reduce effectiveness and cause skin irritation.

To ensure you're using real frankincense, look for products labeled as "pure Boswellia carteri" or "Boswellia sacra" oil. These are the most potent and beneficial types. Reputable brands will often provide information about sourcing and extraction. If you can, choose certified organic frankincense oil to avoid harmful pesticides or chemicals.

How to Use Frankincense in Your Skincare Routine

Incorporating real frankincense into your skincare routine can be simple and highly effective. Here are a few ways to get started:

1. *Facial Serum:* Add a few drops of pure frankincense oil to your regular facial serum or moisturizer. This can enhance the product's ability to hydrate and rejuvenate your skin.

2. *DIY Face Mask:* Mix frankincense oil with honey and yogurt for a soothing and hydrating face mask. Apply it to your face

and leave it on for 15-20 minutes before rinsing off with warm water.

3. *Spot Treatment:* Use frankincense oil as a spot treatment for acne or blemishes. Its anti-inflammatory and antiseptic properties can help reduce redness and speed up healing.

4. *Massage Oil:* Combine frankincense oil with a carrier oil, like jojoba or almond oil, for a luxurious massage blend. This can help improve skin elasticity and reduce the appearance of scars and stretch marks.

Black Seed Oil: Rich and Restorative

From the Nigella sativa plant, black seed oil is a healing powerhouse packed with thymoquinone, an antioxidant that helps calm inflammation and maintain the skin's barrier. This oil is perfect for boosting your skin's natural glow and tackling issues like acne, thanks to its unique blend of fatty acids and vitamins.

Tea Tree Oil: Deep Clean and Clear

Tea tree oil, from the leaves of Melaleuca alternifolia, is renowned for its ability to clear acne-prone skin. Its antibacterial properties penetrate deep to rebalance skin and reduce blemishes, making it a top choice for those seeking a natural approach to achieving clear skin.

Witch Hazel: Gentle, Effective Purity

Witch Hazel, from the Hamamelis virginiana plant, is a natural astringent (skin tissue constrictor) that tightens pores and soothes irritation. It's perfect for oily and acne-prone skin, helping to keep things clear and calm without any harshness.

Bakuchiol: Botanical Balm for Ageless Beauty

Bakuchiol, from the Psoralea corylifolia plant, offers similar benefits to retinol but without the irritation. It fights fine lines, wrinkles, and uneven skin tone, promoting a youthful complexion naturally.

Integrating these natural oils into your skincare routine means you'll be nurturing your skin with the finest that nature has to offer. Each oil has special properties that support skin health and beauty, helping you achieve a clearer, more radiant look.

Chapter 5: Key Takeaways

- **Castor Oil:** Rich in ricinoleic acid, this ancient emollient provides seals in moisture, keeping skin hydrated and supple.
- **Black Seed Oil:** Derived from Nigella sativa seeds, this oil is packed with thymoquinone and unique fatty acids that nourish and heal the skin.
- **Tea Tree Oil:** Known for its antibacterial and anti-inflammatory properties, Tea Tree oil is a powerful remedy for acne and skin irritation.
- **Witch Hazel:** This natural astringent refines pores, soothes inflammation, and balances skin pH.
- **Bakuchiol:** A botanical alternative to retinol, Bakuchiol provides anti-inflammatory and antioxidant benefits.
- **Natural Topicals:** Embracing these oils and extracts maintains skin's balance, health, and radiance without harsh chemicals.

Healthy Skin from Within: The Natural Path to Radiance

Chapter 6: Living in Harmony with Nature

"Create the highest grandest vision possible for your life, because you become what you believe." – Oprah Winfrey

Clean Living Strategies: Clearing the Air and More

Living in a world full of unseen pollutants can silently affect our health, especially our skin. In this chapter, we will recognize these contaminants and find ways to protect ourselves.

Many people don't realize how much their skin contacts daily that impacts their health. I call these "silent toxic killers." North America allows many chemicals in products that are banned elsewhere, so it's crucial to start checking ingredients.

Begin with household cleaning items. Think about what you use to clean your house and dishes. For example, toxins in dishwasher liquids and tablets are endocrine disruptors and are banned in many countries but still used here.

Even new clothes can be covered in toxic chemicals from manufacturing. Always wash new clothes thoroughly before wearing them. Consider adding natural agents like vinegar and baking soda to your laundry.

Many detergents and air fresheners contain chemicals linked to cancer, heart problems, and skin issues. These often include endocrine disruptors. Read the ingredients on all products you use on your body, like body wash, shampoo, conditioner, and face wash. Opt for products with natural ingredients and avoid those with long lists of unpronounceable chemicals.

Air Pollution

Airborne particulates and toxic gasses pose a major threat to skin health, contributing to issues like acne and premature aging. Studies, like those by Fuks et al. (2019), show that air pollution triggers oxidative stress and inflammation in the skin, speeding up damage and aging.

Hormonal Disruptors

Commonly used in agriculture, chemicals like pesticides can disrupt hormonal balance and lead to skin issues such as acne, especially in women (Dreno et al., 2019). Minimizing exposure to these substances can greatly benefit your skin health.

Mold

Often unseen, mold in homes can release mycotoxins that are harmful when inhaled. These toxins can trigger health issues like respiratory problems and skin irritation. This highlights the need for effective mold detection and eradication.

Household Irritants

Everyday products like cleaners, air fresheners, and detergents often contain chemicals that can irritate the skin. A 2009 study (Magnano et al.) linked these chemicals to a higher risk of contact dermatitis. Choosing natural, skin-friendly alternatives can help reduce these risks.

Water Quality

The water we use daily can significantly affect our skin. Contaminants like chlorine and heavy metals strip the skin of natural oils, causing dryness and irritation. Metals like lead and mercury can contribute to oxidative stress, potentially leading to serious skin conditions, including cancer.

Proactive Environmental Management

Reducing exposure to environmental toxins is essential for maintaining skin health and overall well-being. Effective strategies include:

- **Air Filtration:** Use high-quality air purifiers to reduce indoor pollution.
- **Dietary Choices**: Consume antioxidant-rich foods to combat oxidative damage.
- **Natural Cleaning Products**: Opt for fragrance-free, natural cleaning solutions to decrease irritants.
- **Skin Cleansing Routine:** Regularly cleanse your skin to remove pollutants.
- **Water Filtration**: Employ quality water

filters to remove harmful contaminants from your water.

Empowering Choices for Healthier Living

Understanding and managing environmental toxins is key to keeping your skin healthy and boosting your overall vitality. Start by identifying sources of pollutants and then work on limiting your exposure. Make informed choices about what you consume and the products you use. By doing this, you can significantly improve your skin health and energy levels. Remember, reducing toxin exposure is a crucial step toward a healthier you.

Chapter 6: Key Takeaways

- **Air Pollution**: Air pollutants cause oxidative stress and inflammation, leading to premature aging and acne. Use air purifiers and cleanse your skin regularly to reduce these effects.
- **Hormonal Disruptors**: Pesticides and herbicides disrupt hormone balance,

affecting skin health. Eat organic produce and use natural cleaning products to minimize exposure.

- **Mold**: Invisible mold can cause respiratory issues and skin irritation. Regular cleaning and proper ventilation prevent mold growth.
- **Household Product Irritants**: Many household products contain skin irritants. Choose natural, fragrance-free cleaning solutions to avoid reactions.
- **Water Contaminants**: Chlorine and heavy metals in water strip skin of natural oils, causing dryness and irritation. Use quality water filters to improve skin health.
- **Dietary Adjustments**: A diet rich in antioxidants combats oxidative stress from pollutants, supporting skin health.
- **Natural Cleaning Solutions**: Using natural, fragrance-free cleaners reduces exposure to skin irritants.
- **Regular Skin Cleansing**: Cleanse your skin regularly to remove pollutants and reduce the impact of environmental toxins.

- **Water Filtration Methods**: Select effective water filters like Reverse Osmosis or Activated Carbon to remove contaminants and improve skin health.

CHAPTER 7: ANCIENT WISDOM FOR MODERN SKIN

"Nature does not hurry, yet everything is accomplished." - Lao Tzu

Traditional Practices Revisited: Water, Copper, and Quartz for Skin Health

Staying hydrated is key to keeping your skin looking vibrant and healthy. It helps keep your skin supple, supports detoxification, and ensures your cells function properly. This section explores traditional and modern ways to enhance your hydration and keep your skin nourished.

Water: The Foundation of Life

Water is vital for keeping your skin resilient and hydrated. Proper hydration can smooth out fine lines, give your skin a radiant glow, and help flush toxins from your system. Here are some fun ways to increase your water intake:

- **Infuse Your Water:** Add slices of fruits

like lemon or cucumber, or herbs like mint to make it more appealing and encourage drinking.

- **Herbal Teas:** Enjoy hydrating herbal teas like chamomile or peppermint, which offer hydration plus a boost of antioxidants.
- **Monitor Your Intake:** Keep a log of your water intake to make sure you're drinking enough throughout the day.

Coconut Water

Coconut water is full of electrolytes that help maintain fluid balance and support muscle function. It's a delicious, natural way to stay hydrated and feels like a treat with every sip.

Enhanced Hydration with Salt

Adding a pinch of flaky salt to your water can improve hydration efficiency. The salt helps balance electrolytes and increase water absorption at the cellular level.

Chia Seeds: Slow-Release Hydration

Chia seeds can absorb a lot of water and create a gel that slowly releases moisture. Adding them to your water enriches your hydration levels, and even better, provides omega-3 fatty acids and fiber.

Lemon and Baking Soda: Alkalizing Drink

A squeeze of lemon adds vitamin C, and a pinch of baking soda balances pH levels, making for an invigorating, health-boosting drink.

Cucumber and Watermelon: Juicy Additions

Adding cucumber or watermelon to your water boosts electrolytes and nutrients, thanks to their high water content, making hydration tastier and more effective.

Mindful Hydration Tips

- **Room Temperature Water**: Drink water at room temperature for better absorption.
- **Sip Slowly**: Spread out your water intake

throughout the day for more effective hydration.

- **Combine with Fiber**: Eating water-rich fruits and vegetables helps with water absorption.

Copper Vessels

Storing water in copper vessels is an ancient practice with significant health benefits. Copper has antimicrobial properties, enhances digestion, supports skin elasticity, and helps fight free radicals, all contributing to healthier, more youthful skin (Sudha et al., 2012).

Quartz Crystals: Energizing Water

While still under scientific review, many believe that storing water with quartz crystals can purify and revitalize it, potentially enhancing its benefits. This practice connects you with natural elements, boosting your health and overall well-being.

Elements and Their Impact on Skin

Grounding: Connecting with the Earth

Grounding, or earthing, is all about walking barefoot on natural surfaces like grass or sand to soak up the Earth's energy. It's super simple and has been shown to reduce inflammation, boost circulation, and improve skin health. To get started, just find a quiet spot outside, kick off your shoes, and connect your bare feet with the ground for about 20-30 minutes daily. You can enhance this practice by adding some deep breathing to maximize the benefits for glowing, healthy skin.

Sunlight: Harnessing the Power of Natural Light

Moderate sunlight exposure is key for vitamin D production, which is essential for skin health and hormonal balance. To safely enjoy the sun, aim for early morning or late afternoon when the sunlight is gentler. Gradually increase your time in the sun to build your skin's natural resilience and soak up the benefits of natural light while avoiding overexposure.

Natural Sun Protection and Antioxidant-Rich Foods

Protecting your skin from the sun is super important. Go for natural sunscreens that use minerals like zinc oxide or titanium dioxide to create a physical barrier against UV rays. Conventional sunscreens often have chemicals like oxybenzone and octinoxate, which can be harmful. These ingredients can disrupt hormones, cause skin irritation, and even increase the risk of skin cancer. While they're allowed in North America, they're banned in other places like Europe and Asia because of their harmful effects.

Along with using a good sunscreen, eat foods rich in antioxidants to protect against UV damage. Include nutrients like astaxanthin, polyphenols, and omega-3 fatty acids in your diet to help defend against sunburn and boost overall skin health. These steps protect your skin from harmful UV rays and also nourish and support it from the inside out.

The Benefits and Risks of Sun Exposure

Sunlight is not entirely the enemy. In fact,

moderate sun exposure can be beneficial for your skin and overall health. The sun helps your body produce vitamin D, which is crucial for bone health, immune function, and mood regulation. After exposing your skin and eyes to sunlight first thing in the morning, apply a natural, safe sunscreen to protect your skin from prolonged UV radiation.

It's also important to consider the timing and method of your sun protection. Studies have shown that wearing sunglasses can actually increase the likelihood of sunburn. This is because your eyes play a role in signaling to your body how much sun exposure you are getting. Instead of sunglasses, wear a wide-brimmed hat to protect your face while allowing your eyes to receive natural light.

Understanding the Risks of Conventional Sunscreens

Many conventional sunscreens contain chemicals banned in other countries due to health risks. Ingredients like oxybenzone, octinoxate, and homosalate can act as endocrine disruptors, causing hormonal imbalances and other health issues. These chemicals can also contribute to premature aging and skin irritation.

In North America, many of these harmful ingredients are still allowed, so it's crucial to be careful about what you put on your skin. Choose mineral-based sunscreens free from harmful chemicals to ensure you're truly protecting your skin.

Additional Sun Protection Tips

To further protect your skin and enhance your sun protection routine, consider the following tips:

- Wear protective clothing, such as long-sleeved shirts and wide-brimmed hats, especially during peak sunlight hours.
- Seek shade whenever possible, particularly between 10 a.m. and 4 p.m. when the sun's rays are strongest.
- Hydrate your skin from the inside out by drinking plenty of water and consuming foods rich in antioxidants, which can help protect your skin from UV damage.

Chapter 7: Key Takeaways

- **Hydration is Key**: Water is essential for plump, resilient skin and reducing fine lines. Add fruits, herbs, or chia seeds to boost hydration and get extra health benefits.
- **Nature's Sports Drink**: Coconut water is a great natural hydration booster, packed with electrolytes to maintain fluid balance and muscle function.
- **Salt-Infused Water**: Adding a pinch of salt to your water can improve hydration by balancing electrolytes and enhancing water absorption.
- **Copper Vessels**: Storing water in copper vessels adds antimicrobial properties and essential minerals, offering a traditional method for purifying and enhancing water.
- **Quartz Crystals**: Some believe storing water with quartz crystals can purify and revitalize it, potentially boosting overall well-being.
- **Grounding Practice**: Walking barefoot on grass or sand helps reduce inflammation and improve circulation,

leading to healthier, glowing skin.

- **Mindful Sun Exposure**: Moderate sunlight is necessary for vitamin D, but balance it with protective measures like natural sunscreens and antioxidant-rich foods.
- **Natural Sunscreens**: Mineral-based sunscreens provide a physical barrier against UV rays without the harsh chemicals in conventional products.
- **Antioxidant-Rich Foods**: Eating foods high in antioxidants like astaxanthin, polyphenols, and omega-3s enhances the skin's defense against UV damage.

CHAPTER 8: MOVEMENT AND REST

"Walking is man's best medicine" - Hippocrates

Exercise for Skin Health: Best Practices and Routines

When aiming for radiant skin, we often forget how important movement and rest are for our overall well-being. Regular exercise, combined with enough sleep, works wonders in revitalizing your skin from the inside out, boosting your vitality and glow. In this chapter, we'll dive into effective exercises for skin health and the benefits of syncing your workout routines with your menstrual cycle.

The Importance of Weight Training

Weight training offers so many health benefits that shouldn't be underestimated. I've noticed that many women, regardless of age, focus more on cardio. While cardio is great, adding just two 20-minute weightlifting sessions a week can make a huge difference. I remember my trainer pointing out that women who only do cardio often lack muscle tone. Simply by adding weight training, you can slim down, lose inches, and drop body fat more effectively. This means you're getting stronger, improving your overall health, and feeling more confident in your skin. Win-win! Plus, lifting weights boosts circulation and promotes the renewal of skin cells, improving your skin's elasticity and firmness.

My Personal Workout Routine

I've found that 20 minutes of weight lifting is just right for me; any longer can trigger a histamine reaction. Doing this three to four times a week gives me great results. I alternate two exercises at a time, doing 3 sets each with no rest, for a total of 6 different exercises. The time flies by! This structure causes less inflammation in my body compared to extensive cardio or HIIT. Keeping it short and sweet fits better into a busy schedule and avoids overexerting your body and skin.

Exercise and Autoimmune Disorders

If you're dealing with any autoimmune disorder or inflammatory issues, it's important to be aware of how different exercises can affect your body. Studies show that certain types of exercise, especially heavy weightlifting, can raise cortisol levels and potentially worsen these conditions. This doesn't apply to everyone, but it's something to keep in mind, especially for women. Paying attention to your body's signals and adjusting your workout routine accordingly can make a big difference.

Syncing Workouts with Your Menstrual Cycle

One of the best ways to optimize your workouts is by syncing them with your menstrual cycle. In her book "Biohack Like A Woman," Aggie Lal talks about the benefits of exercising according to your hormonal changes throughout the month. For example, during the first few days of your period, it's better to focus on gentle activities like Pilates. As you move into other phases of your cycle, you'll find that you're stronger and can handle more intense weightlifting sessions. Tailoring your workouts to your hormonal cycle can help reduce cortisol levels and inflammation, leading to better results and improved well-being. As Aggie Lal discusses, here's how you can align your exercise routine with your menstrual cycle:

- **Menstrual Phase**: Opt for gentle activities like yoga or light walking during this time to ease cramps and stress while supporting hormonal balance and skin health.
- **Follicular Phase:** As your energy levels increase, ramp up the intensity. This phase is ideal for boosting circulation and collagen production, enhancing your skin's natural radiance.
- **Ovulatory Phase**: Leverage your peak energy to engage in high-intensity workouts. This improves blood flow and detoxification, crucial for maintaining clear skin.
- **Luteal Phase**: You might feel more fatigued as progesterone levels rise. Focus on stress-relieving and low-impact exercises to encourage relaxation and reduce inflammation.

Adapting Your Routine

Being mindful of when and how you exercise, especially around your menstrual cycle, can really boost your workout benefits. It helps lower cortisol levels, reduce inflammation, and avoid insulin resistance, which can cause weight gain. It's all about finding the balance and routine that works best for you. Listen to your body, stay consistent, and enjoy the journey to better health and glowing skin.

Exercises to Enhance Skin Health

Incorporating regular exercise into your daily life is key to maintaining not only a healthy body but also vibrant skin. Here's how different exercises can boost your skin's health:

- **Yoga and Pilates:** More than just stretches, yoga is a full-body approach to wellness that boosts circulation and reduces stress, promoting a healthy glow and inner calm.
- **Swimming**: Dive into the refreshing benefits of water. Swimming is a superb low-impact exercise that helps cleanse

your skin and supports lymphatic drainage, aiding in detoxification and reducing puffiness.

- **Brisk Walking:** A simple yet powerful way to enhance circulation and promote the removal of toxins through sweat, leading to a healthy, glowing complexion.
- **HIIT**: High-Intensity Interval Training boosts circulation and cellular renewal, fighting inflammation and revitalizing the skin.
- **Resistance Training**: It's not just about building muscle strength; resistance training also boosts collagen production, essential for maintaining skin elasticity and reducing signs of aging.

The Role of Sleep

"Sleep is the best meditation." – Dalai Lama

Sleep isn't just rest time; it's when our bodies repair and rejuvenate, keeping our skin youthful and vibrant. At night, our skin cells fix daytime damage and get ready for the next day. Research shows that regular sleep is vital for skin health—lack of sleep can worsen acne, cause dark circles, and speed up aging. Prioritizing sleep is key to supporting your skin's natural repair processes and maintaining a glowing appearance.

Creating a Sleep Sanctuary

To achieve restorative sleep, turn your bedroom into a peaceful, dark, and comfy sanctuary. Invest in quality blackout curtains to keep it dark and consider a white noise machine to block out any noise. A comfortable mattress is also key for a good night's sleep.

Keeping a regular sleep schedule helps align with your body's natural rhythms, promoting deeper, more restorative sleep. Staying consistent, even on weekends, is vital for enhancing skin health and overall vitality.

Minimizing Blue Light Exposure Before Bed

Reduce exposure to blue light from screens before bedtime, as it can disrupt sleep by inhibiting melatonin production. Create a pre-sleep routine free from electronic devices—try a warm bath, reading a book, or doing gentle stretches. This routine signals your body to wind down, making it easier to fall into deep sleep. No need to count sheep!

Managing Stress for Better Sleep

Stress and anxiety, so common in modern life, can really mess with your sleep and, by extension, your skin health. These hidden stressors can worsen skin issues and slow down healing. To help, integrate stress-reducing practices into your nightly routine, like mindfulness meditation, progressive muscle relaxation, or deep breathing exercises.

Nature's Own Sleep Supplements

Quality sleep is essential for glowing skin and overall well-being. Luckily, nature provides many gentle and effective ways to improve sleep. Here are some natural sleep aids backed by science to help you unwind and drift into peaceful slumber.

Saffron

Known mostly for its culinary uses, saffron also has properties that can help you sleep better. It increases the availability of serotonin, a neurotransmitter crucial for regulating sleep. Harvested from the Crocus sativus flower, saffron contains compounds that gently soothe the nervous system, setting the stage for a good night's rest.

Lemon Balm

Lemon balm, with its calming scent and effects, has been a favorite in traditional medicine for ages. It's great for improving sleep quality, especially for those with mild sleep issues. Through promoting relaxation and helping the mind ease into a restful state, lemon balm makes it easier to drift off to sleep.

Valerian Root

Valerian root, known for its sedative qualities, has been used as a sleep aid for centuries. It helps you fall asleep faster and improves sleep quality. Valerian interacts with GABA, a neurotransmitter that regulates nerve impulses in your brain and nervous system, providing a natural sedative effect without the grogginess that often comes with sleep medications.

Suntheanine® (L-theanine): The Relaxation Amino Acid

L-theanine, an amino acid mainly found in green tea, is great for a restful night. Suntheanine®, a patented form of pure L-theanine, has been shown to alter brain wave activity, promoting a state of calm alertness. As it influences GABA levels, it gently encourages relaxation, setting the stage for restorative sleep.

Chapter 8: Key Takeaways

- **Exercise Boosts Skin Health**: Regular activities like yoga, swimming, walking, HIIT, and resistance training improve circulation and detoxification, leading to healthier, more vibrant skin.
- **Match Workouts with Menstrual Cycle**: Align your exercise routine with your menstrual cycle phases for optimal skin health and overall well-being.
- **Restorative Sleep for Skin Repair**: Adequate sleep is crucial for skin repair and rejuvenation, reducing signs of aging and promoting a radiant complexion.
- **Create a Sleep Sanctuary**: Make your

bedroom a cozy, dark, and peaceful space to enhance sleep quality and improve your skin's health.

- **Mindful Sun Exposure**: Get moderate sunlight for vitamin D, but balance it with protective measures like natural sunscreens and antioxidant-rich foods.
- **Natural Sleep Aids**: Use natural sleep supplements like saffron, lemon balm, valerian root, and Suntheanine® to promote restful sleep and healthier skin.
- **Hydration Matters**: Stay hydrated by infusing water with fruits or drinking coconut water to maintain plump, resilient skin.

CHAPTER 9: THE MIND-SKIN CONNECTION

"Mindfulness isn't difficult; we just need to remember to do it." - Sharon Salzberg

Stress and Skin: Understanding and Mitigating Impact

Our mental well-being deeply influences our physical health, especially our skin. Taking care of our emotional and mental health is just as important as any skincare routine or diet we follow.

Stress and Skin: A Troubling Connection

Stress is a common part of life, but it can have profound effects on our skin. When we're stressed, our body releases cortisol, a hormone that disrupts the skin's natural balance. This can lead to inflammation, making conditions like acne, eczema, and psoriasis worse, and weakening the skin's protective barrier. The result is skin that looks as troubled as we feel

178

inside.

Wearing Stress on Our Faces

I've come to realize that I literally wear my stress on my face. I recently read a study that found women who care for children with developmental issues age 6 to 9 years faster on average than those who don't. This really hit home for me because stress can age your skin. My own experience has shown that my mindset directly impacts how fast I age from the inside out. When I'm stressed, I break out more, and stress lines become more noticeable because I frown more. It's taken me years to understand just how important it is to address stress for the sake of my skin health.

Finding Calm to Clear the Skin

Managing stress effectively starts with building inner peace and resilience. Practices like meditation and deep breathing can significantly reduce cortisol levels, soothing inflammation and restoring balance to the skin. These calming practices help us pause, reflect, and manage stress better, preventing the chemical reactions that damage our skin. If I could turn back time, I would have focused not just on nutrition and supplements but also on managing my stress through deep breathing, meditation, gratitude, and manifestation. Making time for self-care has shown immediate results in how I feel and look.

The Healing Power of Sleep

Sleep is when our body and mind repair themselves. During this time, our skin enters a regeneration phase, healing from daily damage. Lack of sleep, often caused by stress, robs us of this crucial recovery time, leaving our skin dull and lifeless. Prioritizing quality sleep and creating a calming bedtime routine can dramatically improve skin health, giving you a refreshed appearance every morning.

Balancing Emotions for Skin Health

Our emotions directly affect our skin health. Stress, sadness, and anger can trigger inflammatory responses in the skin. Developing emotional regulation skills, such as journaling, therapy, or engaging in hobbies, helps maintain both our mental health and our skin's health. When our emotions are balanced, our skin reflects this, appearing healthy and vibrant.

Supporting the Mind-Body-Skin Connection

Getting beautiful skin takes a holistic approach that includes your mind, body, and spirit. Stress-management practices like yoga, tai chi, or just taking daily walks can help align these aspects and promote inner calm, which shows on the outside. Your diet is super important too; eating foods rich in antioxidants and omega-3 fatty acids can counteract the effects of stress on your skin and give you the essential nutrients for optimal skin health.

The Power of Positivity

Maintaining a positive mindset is key to healthier skin. Our thoughts can impact our physical health, and a positive outlook boosts overall well-being, including skin quality. Embracing gratitude and optimism creates a stress-free environment where our skin can flourish. Practicing gratitude every morning and evening, and carrying those positive feelings throughout the day, can significantly lower stress levels and improve your skin.

Mindfulness and Meditation: Tools for Clarity and Glow

Meditation is more than just a mental exercise; it's a powerful tool for skincare. Regular meditation can lower cortisol levels, the stress hormone that often worsens skin conditions like acne and eczema. Starting your day with mindfulness or loving-kindness meditation sets a positive tone, soothing both your mind and skin. This daily practice can lead to clearer, more vibrant skin by keeping you calm throughout the day.

Yoga: Enhancing Circulation and Skin Vitality

Yoga is a holistic practice that combines physical postures, breathing exercises, and meditation to manage stress and improve skin health. As you move through yoga poses, you boost blood flow, ensuring your skin gets essential nutrients. Yoga also helps eliminate toxins that can cause blemishes. Adding both gentle and dynamic yoga sequences to your routine can support a balanced mind and glowing skin.

Journaling: Emotional Release for Skin Clarity

Journaling is a therapeutic tool that gives you a private space to express your thoughts and emotions. Regularly writing down your feelings can help relieve emotional stress that might trigger skin flare-ups. This daily practice offers a safe outlet for emotional release, leading to healthier, more resilient skin.

Deep Breathing: Infusing Oxygen into Your Skin

Deep breathing is a simple yet effective way to boost your skin's health. Taking deep, controlled breaths increases oxygen uptake, vital for cell health and skin regeneration. Use deep breathing techniques during stressful moments to reduce their impact on your skin, preventing stress-induced skin issues.

Progressive Muscle Relaxation: Smoothing the Skin

Stress often shows up as muscle tension, which can negatively affect your skin. Progressive muscle relaxation, where you tense and then relax each muscle group, can help alleviate physical stress and improve blood circulation. Better circulation delivers more nutrients to skin cells, helping with repair and resilience against damage.

Guided Imagery: Visualizing Healthier Skin

Guided imagery involves visualizing calming and healing scenarios, which can be especially helpful for those with skin issues. If you spend time imagining your skin healing and glowing, you nurture a positive mindset that can influence your body's healing processes. This practice helps to encourage a positive outlook and healthier skin through the power of visualization.

The Power of Gratitude and Manifestation

Gratitude is so powerful for your mental and emotional well-being, and will also benefit your skin. Start each day by listing things you're grateful for regarding your health and skin journey, no matter how small. This simple practice shifts your focus from what's wrong to what's right, reducing stress and promoting a sense of well-being. Keep this gratitude mindset throughout the day and revisit it in the evening, reflecting on the positive aspects of your life. This continuous focus on gratitude can significantly lower stress levels, which is directly linked to healthier skin.

Manifestation is another powerful tool. Imagine all your skin goals came true yesterday. How would you feel? What activities would you be enjoying? For example, if you had clear skin, maybe you'd book a professional photoshoot. Spend time each evening writing down these feelings and activities as if they are already your reality. This practice boosts your mood and helps lower stress levels, creating a healthier environment for your skin to thrive. Carry these positive feelings into your daily life, and you can manifest any reality you want, improving your overall health and skin condition.

Combining Mindfulness, Gratitude, and Manifestation

Start your morning by listing things you're

grateful for, no matter how small. Then, try some guided imagery by visualizing your skin healing and glowing. Picture yourself doing activities that make you happy and fulfilled. Keep this positive mindset going throughout the day. In the evening, write down your feelings and experiences as if your dreams have already come true.

Combining mindfulness, gratitude, and manifestation boosts your mental and emotional well-being while also helping your skin look healthier and more vibrant. These techniques reduce stress and promote a positive outlook. Guided imagery lets you see your desired outcome, while gratitude and manifestation keep you focused on positive feelings. This combo can transform your mindset, lower stress levels, and directly improve your skin health.

Chapter 9: Key Takeaways

- **Stress-Skin Connection**: Stress releases cortisol, upsetting skin balance and causing inflammation, acne, or eczema. Calming practices can improve skin health.

- **Meditation for Skin Health**: Regular meditation lowers cortisol levels, leading to clearer, more radiant skin. Incorporate mindfulness or loving-kindness meditation into your daily routine.
- **Yoga's Dual Benefits**: Yoga boosts blood circulation and detoxification, delivering nutrients to the skin and clearing away toxins. Relaxing and energizing poses promote a calm mind and glowing complexion.
- **Journaling for Emotional Release**: Writing down thoughts and feelings helps relieve emotional stress, which can cause skin problems. Daily journaling lightens emotional burdens and leads to healthier skin.
- **Deep Breathing for Oxygenation**: Deep breathing exercises increase oxygen flow to the skin, promoting cell health and regeneration. This practice instantly relieves stress and benefits the skin.
- **Progressive Muscle Relaxation**: Tension in the body can worsen skin issues. Progressive muscle relaxation reduces physical stress and improves blood

circulation, aiding skin health and resilience.

- **Guided Imagery**: Visualizing healing and positive images can influence the body's healing process and improve skin conditions. This practice promotes a positive mindset and skin healing.

CHAPTER 10: TOWARD SUSTAINABLE BEAUTY

"We do not inherit the earth from our ancestors; we borrow it from our children." – Native American Proverb

Eco-Friendly Skincare: Choosing Wisely for Ourselves and the Planet

In today's world, where environmental challenges are front and center, the beauty industry has a huge role in promoting sustainability. Choosing sustainable and eco-friendly skincare, whether it's something you apply or ingest, is a way to commit to the planet and future generations. When we opt for products that are gentle on both our skin and the environment, we're supporting a bigger movement to preserve and respect our natural world.

Core Values of Sustainable Skincare Brands

Sustainable skincare and wellness companies are leading an eco-conscious revolution, showing that beauty and environmental care can go hand in hand. These pioneers follow a few fundamental principles:

- **Natural and Organic Ingredients**: These brands focus on eco-friendly sourcing, using natural and organic materials that avoid harmful chemicals, benefiting both our skin and the planet.

- **Green Manufacturing Practices**: Eco-conscious companies use sustainable production methods, invest in renewable energy, and prioritize efficient resource use to reduce their ecological footprint.

- **Cruelty-Free and Vegan Products**: Ethical skincare brands ensure no animals are harmed during production. They advocate for cruelty-free testing and offer vegan options, aligning with compassionate values.

- **Sustainable Packaging**: These companies use minimal, recyclable, or biodegradable packaging, and explore refillable options to reduce waste and support a circular economy.

- **Community and Environmental Engagement**: Many sustainable brands actively support community and environmental initiatives, like tree planting, clean water projects, and wildlife conservation, showing their commitment to the planet.

Empowering Consumers With The Power of Choice

As consumers, our choices make a big difference. Picking eco-friendly products means caring for our skin and supporting a sustainable future. It's important to be informed, understand ingredient impacts, and choose products that reflect our values. With this approach, we're partnering with brands to create a greener, more sustainable world. Let's make those choices together for a better planet!

Innovations in Sustainable Skincare

The future of sustainable skincare looks bright. Brands are always finding new ways to reduce their environmental impact, like creating biodegradable formulas and using energy-efficient processes. The rise of zero-waste products and upcycled materials shows promising trends towards more eco-friendly practices. As technology and environmental awareness grow, we can expect even more innovative solutions in sustainable beauty.

A Collective Effort for a Greener Planet

Choosing eco-friendly skincare is a step towards a better, more sustainable planet. Supporting eco-friendly practices in the beauty industry means we're helping to ensure that the beauty we enjoy today can be appreciated by future generations. The journey to radiant skin and a healthy planet is in our hands, and together, we can make a big impact. Let's do our part and make a difference!

Reducing Waste: Tips and Strategies for Conscious Living

Choosing sustainable skincare brands is a great first step. Look for companies that focus on ethical sourcing, use green manufacturing processes, and engage in environmental conservation. These brands use natural and organic ingredients and work to minimize their environmental impact. By choosing these products, you're caring for your skin and helping the planet.

Simplifying Your Routine with Multi-Functional Products

Embracing a minimalist skincare approach doesn't mean compromising on quality or effectiveness. It's about choosing multi-functional products that meet your skin's true needs, reducing the number of products you use. This strategy cuts down on waste and can save you time and money. Look for products that offer hydration, protection, and nourishment all in one, and those that combine makeup with skincare benefits.

Making Smart Packaging Choices

Packaging is a big waste contributor in skincare. Go for products with minimal packaging or ones using recycled, recyclable, or biodegradable materials. Many brands offer refillable options, cutting down on waste over time. Buying in bulk can also reduce how often you need to buy and the packaging waste that comes with it.

Repurposing and Recycling

Before tossing them out, think about repurposing your skincare containers. Glass jars can hold small items, and pump bottles can be reused for your own skincare creations. If you can't repurpose, make sure to recycle correctly. Check your local recycling guidelines, as some materials need special handling. Some companies even offer take-back programs to ensure packaging is recycled or disposed of responsibly.

Streamlining Your Skincare Collection

A cluttered skincare shelf can lead to waste. Streamline your routine by using up products before buying new ones and resisting every new trend. This way, you fully utilize each product and get to know what works best for your skin. Remember, a product only benefits your skin if you actually use it, not if it just sits on your shelf.

Advocacy and Education

Stay informed about the beauty industry's environmental impact and share what you learn. Advocating for sustainability can prompt more brands to adopt eco-friendly practices. Join online forums, community discussions, and support organizations promoting sustainable beauty. Your voice can inspire others, creating a ripple effect that strengthens the movement toward a sustainable future.

Chapter 10: Key Takeaways

- **Eco-Friendly Choices**: Choose skincare products from sustainable brands with eco-conscious practices like ethical sourcing and green manufacturing to help reduce environmental impact.
- **Core Values of Sustainable Brands**: Sustainable brands prioritize natural and organic ingredients, cruelty-free testing, green manufacturing, ethical sourcing, and community engagement.
- **Consumer Power**: Make informed choices by reading labels and understanding ingredients to support

sustainable practices and encourage the industry to go green.

- **Innovations in Sustainability**: The skincare industry is evolving with biodegradable formulas, zero-waste products, and upcycled materials, offering more eco-friendly options.
- **Reducing Waste with Minimalism**: A minimalist skincare routine with multipurpose products helps reduce waste, save money, and simplify daily rituals.
- **Sustainable Packaging**: Choose products with minimal, recycled, recyclable, or biodegradable packaging to reduce waste and environmental footprint.
- **Repurposing and Recycling**: Repurpose old skincare containers and recycle them properly to minimize waste and promote a sustainable lifestyle.
- **Streamlining Skincare**: Use products completely before buying new ones and avoid every new trend to reduce waste and ensure a focused, effective routine.
- **Advocacy and Education**: Stay informed

about the beauty industry's environmental impacts and advocate for sustainable practices to drive larger-scale changes.

- **Sustainable Living**: Embrace sustainability in all aspects of life, including skincare, to reduce our ecological footprint and contribute to a healthier planet for future generations.

Chapter 11: Embracing Your Journey

"Alone, we can do so little; together, we can do so much" – Helen Keller

Community and Support: Finding Strength Together

Sharing this pathway of skin wins with others who understand your goals and challenges can make a big difference. Having a community of like-minded individuals is invaluable. It offers a space to exchange knowledge, share experiences, and boost morale. Whether through online forums, local groups, or social media, connecting with others enriches your perspective on skincare. Finding your tribe means joining a safe, welcoming space where everyone feels comfortable to express their thoughts and learn from each other.

The Strength of Shared Experiences

There's undeniable power in numbers. Sharing your skincare journey can bring emotional support, practical tips, and a sense of belonging. It's about celebrating successes together and offering support during setbacks. Learning from others' experiences can spark new ideas and inspire solutions that might be just what you need. The goal is to share knowledge so the whole community benefits.

Engaging in Educational Events

Get involved in workshops, webinars, and events focused on holistic skincare. These gatherings are perfect for learning from experts, discovering new products, and networking with fellow skincare enthusiasts. Attending these events can expand your understanding and empower you to make better choices for your skin.

Building Accountability Partnerships

Find a skincare buddy and hold each other accountable. Chat about your goals, routines, and progress. Regular check-ins with someone who's cheering you on can really boost your commitment to your skincare routine and help you stay on track.

Sharing Your Story

Consider documenting and sharing your skincare journey. Whether it's through blogging, vlogging, or social media updates, telling your story can inspire and encourage others. Share both the highs and the lows—your honest journey can resonate deeply, offering hope and connection.

Embracing Diversity and Inclusivity

Cultivate a community that celebrates diversity and embraces everyone's unique journey. Remember, everyone's skin is different; what works for one person might not work for another. Valuing diverse perspectives and backgrounds enriches the community and broadens our collective understanding of skincare.

Continuous Learning and Adapting

The world of holistic skincare is always changing! Stay open and curious about new research, products, and techniques. Keep the conversation going and share fresh insights with your community. Being adaptable and open to new information is key to keeping your skincare routine effective and fun.

Continuing Your Path: Practical Advice for Ongoing Care

Embracing a lifetime of glowing, healthy skin means committing to more than just quick fixes. Your skincare approach should be ongoing and adaptable, changing over time to meet your evolving needs and lifestyle.

Consistency and Patience: The Foundations of Skincare Success

The key to any skincare routine is consistency. Regular care is crucial, so establish and stick to a daily regimen. Patience is essential, as visible results can take time. The goal is to support and enhance your skin's natural functions, not to chase an unattainable ideal of perfection.

Adapting to Your Skin's Evolving Needs

As you age, your skin's needs will change due

to hormonal shifts, environmental conditions, and lifestyle choices. Regularly assess your skin's condition and adjust your skincare routine accordingly. Consulting with a dermatologist or skincare professional can provide insights into the best practices and products for your skin's current needs.

A Holistic Approach to Health

As we've learned in this book, beautiful skin reflects your overall health and well-being. Make sure to get enough sleep, drink plenty of water, eat a nutrient-rich diet, and manage stress effectively. These lifestyle choices have a big impact on your skin's health and appearance.

Choosing the Right Products

Navigating the sea of skincare products can be totally overwhelming. Go for ones that are gentle yet effective, as natural as possible, and perfect for your skin type and concerns. Steer clear of harsh chemicals that strip your skin of natural oils or cause irritation. Look for products that support your skin's barrier and keep things balanced.

Embrace Lifelong Skincare Learning

Your journey to healthy, radiant skin is ongoing. Embrace the process of learning and adapting as your skin changes. Celebrate your progress and learn from any setbacks. Keep exploring new practices and products that match your evolving skincare needs and values. This lifelong commitment to learning and adapting is the key to achieving and maintaining vibrant skin.

Chapter 11: Key Takeaways

- **Shared Experiences**: Sharing your skincare journey with others provides emotional support, practical advice, and a sense of camaraderie. It's all about growing and understanding together.
- **Educational Engagement**: Join workshops and events focused on holistic skincare to learn new practices, meet experts, and connect with other enthusiasts.
- **Accountability Partnerships**: Find a skincare buddy to share goals and progress. It keeps you committed and

motivated with mutual encouragement.

- **Embracing Diversity and Inclusivity**: Celebrate the diversity in the skincare community. It enriches collective knowledge and provides a well-rounded understanding of holistic practices.
- **Consistency and Patience**: Stick to a regular skincare routine. Patience is key since results take time to show.
- **Holistic Health Approach**: Healthy skin is tied to overall health. Pay attention to your diet, manage stress, and get enough sleep to maintain skin vitality.
- **Embracing the Journey**: Skincare is a lifelong process. Keep learning, adapting, and appreciating your skin's unique journey.

CONCLUSION

Final Thoughts and Encouragement

In this book, we've explored all the ways to nurture your skin by harmonizing your body, mind, and environment. I hope this guide has helped you embrace a holistic lifestyle that boosts every aspect of your being, showing up as the clear, radiant skin you desire. Remember, your skin journey is personal and ongoing—keep learning, adapting, and celebrating your progress. Here's to a lifetime of glowing, healthy skin!

Embracing a Holistic Approach to Well-being

Your skin reflects your internal health and emotional state. Moving forward, remember that every choice you make, from the food you eat to your thoughts, affects your skin's health. Achieving clear skin is about creating a lifestyle filled with vitality and happiness, not just being acne-free. Balance your diet with nutrient-rich foods, manage stress through mindfulness, and care for your skin with natural, sustainable products. These steps are commitments to a healthier, more vibrant you.

Setting Intentions for a Wholesome Life

As you continue on this path, focus on setting intentions rather than strict rules. Commit to treating your body with love, nourishing your skin with what it needs, and creating a supportive environment for your well-being. Reflect on your habits, understand your body's unique signals, and tailor your routines to meet your skin's evolving needs.

Staying Flexible and Responsive

Your skin and its needs will change over time due to hormonal shifts and environmental factors. Regularly check in on your skin's condition and your overall health. Stay adaptable and be ready to tweak your skincare approach as needed. This ensures your routine stays effective and in tune with your current needs. Keep listening to your skin, and adjust your care to keep it healthy and glowing.

In Conclusion: A Journey Just Beginning

As you close this book, remember your journey is just beginning. Armed with new knowledge and strategies, move forward with confidence and enthusiasm. Every day is a new opportunity to enhance your well-being and skin health. Embrace this journey with the joy and uniqueness it deserves—it's as beautiful and distinct as you are. Here's to glowing skin and a vibrant life!

About the Author

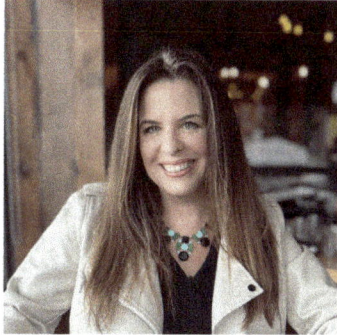

Joanna Bacchus is a pioneer in the nutritional supplements industry. As a Certified Nutritional Advisor and the visionary behind Elsantis and BIOSTRIPS™, Joanna turned her struggles with entrepreneurial and parental exhaustion into an innovative wellness journey. Frustrated by traditional supplements' inefficiencies and chemical-heavy formulations, she spent five years researching and collaborating with top scientists. And along came BIOSTRIPS™—vegan, eco-friendly, and highly bioavailable supplements designed to support busy people at all life stages. Joanna's work highlights her dedication to convenient, effective health solutions, making a significant impact on the supplement market and empowering individuals to easily take charge of their health.

REFERENCES

Archer, D. F. "Menstrual-cycle-related symptoms: a review of the rationale for continuous use of oral contraceptives." Contraception, vol. 74, no. 5, 2004, pp. 359–366.

Aguayo-Morales H, Sierra-Rivera CA, Claudio-Rizo JA, Cobos-Puc LE. Horsetail (Equisetum hyemale) Extract Accelerates Wound Healing in Diabetic Rats by Modulating IL-10 and MCP-1 Release and Collagen Synthesis. Pharmaceuticals (Basel). 2023 Mar 30;16(4):514. doi: 10.3390/ph16040514. PMID: 37111271; PMCID: PMC10141616.

Ali, Mohammad & Rahayu, Setya & Indardi, Nanang & Anggita, Gustiana Mega & Suraya, Fatona & Rustadi, Tri & Wicaksono, Anggit & Chen, Yu & Chang, Yun. (2018). Usage of Fruit-Infused Water for Prevention of Dehydration Due to Endurance Exercise. Jurnal Kesehatan Masyarakat. 13. 417-422. 10.15294/kemas.v13i3.12977.

Araújo LA, Addor F, Campos PM. "Use of silicon for skin and hair care: an approach of chemical forms available and efficacy." An Bras Dermatol. 2016 May-Jun;91(3):331-5. doi: 10.1590/abd1806-4841.20163986. PMID: 27438201; PMCID: PMC4938278.

Bhusal KK, Magar SK, Thapa R, Lamsal A, Bhandari S, Maharjan R, Shrestha S, Shrestha J. Nutritional and pharmacological importance of stinging nettle (Urtica dioica L.): A review. Heliyon. 2022 Jun 22;8(6):e09717. doi: 10.1016/j.heliyon.2022.e09717. PMID: 35800714; PMCID: PMC9253158.

Black HS, Rhodes LE. Potential Benefits of Omega-3 Fatty Acids in Non-Melanoma Skin Cancer. J Clin Med. 2016 Feb 4;5(2):23. doi: 10.3390/jcm5020023. PMID: 26861407; PMCID: PMC4773779.

Bowe, W.P., Logan, A.C. Acne vulgaris,

probiotics and the gut-brain-skin axis - back to the future?. Gut Pathog 3, 1 (2011). https://doi.org/10.1186/1757-4749-3-1

Chandrasekhar, K., et al. "A prospective, randomized double-blind, placebo-controlled study of safety and efficacy of a high-concentration full-spectrum extract of ashwagandha root in reducing stress and anxiety in adults." Indian Journal of Psychological Medicine, vol. 34, no. 3, 2012, pp. 255–262.

Cho S, Lee S, Lee MJ, Lee DH, Won CH, Kim SM, Chung JH. Dietary Aloe Vera Supplementation Improves Facial Wrinkles and Elasticity and It Increases the Type I Procollagen Gene Expression in Human Skin in vivo. Ann Dermatol. 2009 Feb;21(1):6-11. https://doi.org/10.5021/ad.2009.21.1.6

Catherine K. Huang, Timothy A. Miller, The Truth About Over-the-Counter Topical Anti-Aging Products: A Comprehensive Review, Aesthetic Surgery Journal, Volume 27, Issue 4, July 2007, Pages 402–412, https://doi.org/10.1016/j.asj.2007.05.005

Chiu, April E., et al. "The Response of Skin Disease to Stress: Changes in the Severity of Acne Vulgaris as Affected by Examination Stress." Archives of Dermatology, vol. 141, no. 7, 2005, pp. 897–900.

Cosgrove, Maeve C., et al. "Dietary nutrient intakes and skin-aging appearance among middle-aged American women." The American Journal of Clinical Nutrition, vol. 86, no. 4, 2007, pp. 1225–1231.

Daughton CG, Ternes TA. Pharmaceuticals and personal care products in the environment: agents of subtle change? Environ Health Perspect. 1999 Dec;107 Suppl 6(Suppl 6):907-38. doi: 10.1289/ehp.99107s6907. PMID: 10592150; PMCID: PMC1566206.

de Oliveira AP, Franco Ede S, Rodrigues Barreto R, Cordeiro DP, de Melo RG, de Aquino CM, E Silva AA, de Medeiros PL, da Silva TG, Góes AJ, Maia MB. Effect of semisolid formulation of persea americana mill (avocado) oil on wound healing in rats. Evid Based Complement Alternat Med. 2013;2013:472382. doi: 10.1155/2013/472382. Epub 2013 Mar 19. PMID: 23573130; PMCID: PMC3614059.

Dréno B, Bettoli V, Araviiskaia E, Sanchez Viera M, Bouloc A. The influence of exposome on acne. J Eur Acad Dermatol Venereol. 2018 May;32(5):812-819. doi: 10.1111/jdv.14820. Epub 2018 Feb 15. PMID: 29377341; PMCID: PMC5947266.

Ekanayake-Mudiyanselage, S., & Thiele, J. (2006). Vitamin E in Skin Health and Function. In Cosmeceuticals and Active Cosmetics, 2nd Edition (pp. 111-131). CRC Press.

Fuks KB, Hüls A, Sugiri D, Altug H, Vierkötter A, Abramson MJ, Goebel J, Wagner GG, Demuth I, Krutmann J, Schikowski T. Tropospheric ozone and skin aging: Results from two German cohort studies. Environ Int. 2019 Mar;124:139-144. doi: 10.1016/j.envint.2018.12.047. Epub 2019 Jan 11. PMID: 30641257.

Ferruzzi, M.G. & Blakeslee, J., "Digestion,

absorption, and cancer preventative activity of dietary chlorophyll derivatives," Food and Chemical Toxicology, 2007

"Fluoride in Drinking-water". World Health Organization, 2004, pp. 1-144. WHO.

Guo M, Lu Y, Yang J, Zhao X, Lu Y. "Inhibitory effects of Schisandra chinensis extract on acne-related inflammation and UVB-induced photoageing." Pharm Biol. 2016 Dec;54(12):2987-2994. doi: 10.1080/13880209.2016.1199041. Epub 2016 Jun 22. PMID: 27328727.

Gruszczyńska M, Sadowska-Przytocka A, Szybiak W, Więckowska B, Lacka K. Insulin Resistance in Patients with Acne Vulgaris. Biomedicines. 2023 Aug 18;11(8):2294. doi: 10.3390/biomedicines11082294. PMID: 37626790; PMCID: PMC10452885.

Gupta, Madhulika, et al. "Zinc therapy in dermatology: a review." Dermatology Research and Practice, 2014.

Harrison F, Furner-Pardoe J, Connelly E. An assessment of the evidence for antibacterial activity of stinging nettle (Urtica dioica) extracts. Access Microbiol. 2022 Mar 24;4(3):000336. doi: 10.1099/acmi.0.000336. PMID: 35693473; PMCID: PMC9175978.

Hekmatpou, D., 2008. "The Effect of Aloe Vera Gel on Skin Hydration." Skin Pharmacology and Physiology.

Hughes, D. J. (2012). Selenium in health and disease: A review. Critical Reviews in Food Science and Nutrition, 52(4), 360-368. doi: 10.1080/10408398.2010.499819.

Holick, Michael F. "Vitamin D deficiency." New England Journal of Medicine, vol. 357, no. 3, 2007, pp. 266-281.

Jabbar-Lopez ZK, Ung CY, Alexander H, Gurung N, Chalmers J, Danby S, Cork MJ, Peacock JL, Flohr C. The effect of water hardness on atopic eczema, skin barrier function: A systematic review, meta-analysis. Clin Exp Allergy. 2021 Mar;51(3):430-451. doi: 10.1111/cea.13797.

Epub 2020 Dec 13. PMID: 33259122.

Jelena Popović-Djordjević, Bojana Špirović-Trifunović, Ilinka Pećinar, Luiz Fernando Cappa de Oliveira, Đurđa Krstić, Dragana Mihajlović, Milica Fotirić Akšić, Jesus Simal-Gandara, Fatty acids in seed oil of wild and cultivated rosehip (Rosa canina L.) from different locations in Serbia, Industrial Crops and Products, Volume 191, Part B, 2023, 115797, ISSN 0926-6690, https://doi.org/10.1016/j.indcrop.2022.115797.

Jubert, C., et al., "Effects of Chlorophyll and Chlorophyllin on Low-Dose Aflatoxin B1 Pharmacokinetics in Human Volunteers," Journal of Alternative and Complementary Medicine, 2009

Jefferson, Wendy N. "Adult ovarian function can be affected by high levels of soy." The Journal of Nutrition, vol. 140, no. 12, 2010, pp. 2322S-2325S.

Jéquier, E., & Constant, F. (2010). Water as an essential nutrient: the physiological basis of hydration. European Journal of Clinical Nutrition, 64(2), 115–123. doi: 10.1038/ejcn.2009.111. PMID: 19724292.

Keen, M. A., & Hassan, I. (2016). Vitamin E in dermatology. Indian Dermatology Online Journal, 7(4), 311–315. doi: 10.4103/2229-5178.185494.

Keser S, Celik S, Turkoglu S, Yilmaz Ö, Turkoglu I. The investigation of some bioactive compounds and antioxidant properties of hawthorn (Crataegus monogyna subsp. monogyna Jacq). J Intercult Ethnopharmacol. 2014 Apr-Jun;3(2):51-5. doi: 10.5455/jice.20140120103320. Epub 2014 May 23. PMID: 26401347; PMCID: PMC4576801.

Khedmat H, Karbasi A, Amini M, Aghaei A, Taheri S. Aloe vera in treatment of refractory irritable bowel syndrome: Trial on Iranian patients. J Res Med Sci. 2013 Aug;18(8):732. PMID: 24379854; PMCID: PMC3872617.

Kafi, R., Kwak, H. S., Schumacher, W. E., Cho, S., Hanft, V. N., Hamilton, T. A., ... & Kang, S. (2007). Improvement of naturally aged skin with vitamin A (retinol). Archives of Dermatology, 143(5), 606-612. doi: 10.1001/archderm.143.5.606.

Kaczmarczyk, M.M., et al. "The health benefits of dietary fiber: beyond the usual suspects of type 2 diabetes mellitus, cardiovascular disease and colon cancer." Metabolism, vol. 61, no. 8, 2012, pp. 1058-1066.

Katiyar, Santosh K., and Craig A. Elmets. "Green tea polyphenolic antioxidants and skin photoprotection." International Journal of Oncology, vol. 18, no. 6, 2001, pp. 1307–1313.

Kim SJ. Effect of biflavones of Ginkgo biloba against UVB-induced cytotoxicity in vitro. J Dermatol. 2001 Apr;28(4):193-9. doi: 10.1111/j.1346-8138.2001.tb00117.x. PMID: 11449670.

Kumari, Rashmi, et al. "Skin changes in pregnancy: a study of 2000 antenatal patients." Global journal of health science, vol. 7, no. 1, 2015, p. 195.

"Lead In Water: What Are The Health Effects And Dangers?". Popular Science, 2021.

Li Y, Su J, Luo D, Duan Y, Huang Z, He M, Tao J, Xiao S, Xiao Y, Chen X, Shen M. Processed Food and Atopic Dermatitis: A Pooled Analysis of Three Cross-Sectional Studies in Chinese Adults. Front Nutr. 2021 Dec 6;8:754663. doi: 10.3389/fnut.2021.754663. PMID: 34938758; PMCID: PMC8685501.

Liu S, You L, Zhao Y, Chang X. "Hawthorn Polyphenol Extract Inhibits UVB-Induced Skin Photoaging by Regulating MMP Expression and Type I Procollagen Production in Mice." J Agric Food Chem. 2018 Aug 15;66(32):8537-8546. doi: 10.1021/acs.jafc.8b02785. Epub 2018 Jul 31. PMID: 30032605.

Magnano M, Silvani S, Vincenzi C, Nino M, Tosti A. Contact allergens and irritants in household washing and cleaning products. Contact Dermatitis. 2009 Dec;61(6):337-41. doi: 10.1111/j.1600-0536.2009.01647.x. PMID: 20059494.

Merfort I, Heilmann J, Hagedorn-Leweke U, Lippold BC. In vivo skin penetration studies of camomile flavones. Die Pharmazie. 1994 Jul;49(7):509-511. PMID: 8073060.

Meissner, H.O., et al. "Hormone-Balancing Effect of Pre-Gelatinized Organic Maca (Lepidium Peruvianum Chacon): (I) Biochemical and Pharmacodynamic Study on Maca using Clinical Laboratory Model on Ovariectomized Rats." International Journal of Biomedical Science, vol. 2, no. 3, 2006, pp. 260–272.

Mukherjee, S., Date, A., Patravale, V., Korting, H. C., Roeder, A., & Weindl, G. (2006). Retinoids in the treatment of skin aging: an overview of clinical efficacy and safety. Clinical Interventions in Aging, 1(4), 327–348. PMID: 18046911.

Neltner TJ, Sahoo PK, Smith RW, Anders JPV, Arnett JE, Schmidt RJ, Johnson GO, Natarajan SK, Housh TJ. Effects of 8 Weeks of Shilajit Supplementation on Serum Pro-c1α1, a Biomarker of Type 1 Collagen Synthesis: A Randomized Control Trial. J Diet Suppl. 2024;21(1):1-12.   doi:

10.1080/19390211.2022.2157522. Epub 2022 Dec 22. PMID: 36546868.

Phetcharat L, Wongsuphasawat K, Winther K. "The effectiveness of a standardized rose hip powder containing seeds and shells of Rosa canina on cell longevity, skin wrinkles, moisture, and elasticity." Clin Interv Aging. 2015 Nov 19;10:1849-56. doi: 10.2147/CIA.S90092. PMID: 26604725; PMCID: PMC4655903.

Pan, Junying & Wang, Haoyu & Chen, Yinghua. "Prunella vulgaris L. – A Review of its Ethnopharmacology, Phytochemistry, Quality Control and Pharmacological Effects." Frontiers in Pharmacology. 13. 903171. 2022. doi: 10.3389/fphar.2022.903171.

Palma, L., Marques, L. T., Bujan, J., & Rodrigues, L. M. (2015). Dietary water affects human skin hydration and biomechanics. Clinical, Cosmetic and Investigational Dermatology, 8, 413–421. doi: 10.2147/CCID.S86822. PMID: 26345226.

Pappas, Apostolos. "The relationship of diet and acne: A review." Dermatoendocrinology, vol. 1, no. 5, 2009, pp. 262–267.

Penniston, K. L., & Tanumihardjo, S. A. (2006). The acute and chronic toxic effects of vitamin A. The American Journal of Clinical Nutrition, 83(2), 191-201. doi: 10.1093/ajcn/83.2.191.

Popkin, B. M., D'Anci, K. E., & Rosenberg, I. H. (2010). Water, Hydration and Health. Nutrition Reviews, 68(8), 439–458. doi: 10.1111/j.1753-4887.2010.00304.x. PMID: 20646222.

Podda, M., Traber, M. G., & Packer, L. (1999). UV-Irradiation Depletes Antioxidants and Causes Oxidative Damage in a Model of Human Skin. Free Radical Biology and Medicine, 26(1-2), 42-48. doi: 10.1016/S0891-5849(98)00186-8.

Pieroth R, Paver S, Day S, Lammersfeld C. Folate and Its Impact on Cancer Risk. Curr Nutr Rep. 2018 Sep;7(3):70-84. doi: 10.1007/s13668-018-0237-y. PMID: 30099693; PMCID: PMC6132377.

Pullar, Juliet M., et al. "The Roles of Vitamin C in Skin Health." Nutrients, vol. 9, no. 8, 2017, p. 866.

Rao R, Samak G. Role of Glutamine in Protection of Intestinal Epithelial Tight Junctions. J Epithel Biol Pharmacol. 2012 Jan;5(Suppl 1-M7):47-54. doi: 10.2174/1875044301205010047. PMID: 25810794; PMCID: PMC4369670.

Riebl, S. K., & Davy, B. M. (2013). The Hydration Equation: Update on Water Balance and Cognitive Performance. ACSM's Health & Fitness Journal, 17(6), 21–28. doi: 10.1249/FIT.0b013e3182a9570f.

Reichrath, J., Lehmann, B., Carlberg, C., Varani, J., & Zouboulis, C. C. (2007). Vitamins as hormones. Hormone and Metabolic Research, 39(2), 71-84. doi: 10.1055/s-2007-961384.

Szlyk, P., Ingrid V. Sils, Ralph P. Francesconi, Roger W. Hubbard, Lawrence E. Armstrong,

Effects of water temperature and flavoring on voluntary dehydration in men, Physiology & Behavior, Volume 45, Issue 3, 1989, Pages 639-647, ISSN 0031-9384, https://doi.org/10.1016/0031-9384(89)90085-1.

Soleymani, T., Hung, T., & Soung, J. (2015). The role of vitamin D in psoriasis: A review. International Journal of Dermatology, 54(4), 383-392. doi: 10.1111/ijd.12790.

Srivastava JK, Shankar E and Gupta S: Chamomile: A herbal medicine of the past with a bright future (Review). Mol Med Rep 3: 895-901, 2010

Sartori, S.B., et al. "Magnesium deficiency induces anxiety and HPA axis dysregulation: Modulation by therapeutic drug treatment." Neuropharmacology, vol. 62, no. 1, 2012, pp. 304-312.

Semba, R. D. (1999). Vitamin A, immunity, and infection. Clinics in Dermatology, 17(4), 393-399. doi: 10.1016/s0738-081x(99)00046-9.

Sies, Helmut, and Wilhelm Stahl. "Nutritional protection against skin damage from sunlight." Annual Review of Nutrition, vol. 24, 2004, pp. 173–200.

Simopoulos, Artemis P. "The importance of the ratio of omega-6/omega-3 essential fatty acids." Biomedicine & Pharmacotherapy, vol. 56, no. 8, 2002, pp. 365-379.

Simopoulos, Artemis P. "Omega-3 fatty acids in inflammation and autoimmune diseases." Journal of the American College of Nutrition, vol. 21, no. 6, 2002, pp. 495–505.

Shuster, Sam, et al. "The cause and measurement of the menopausal hot flush." British Journal of Pharmacology and Chemotherapy, vol. 55, no. 2, 1975, pp. 157–161.

Sudha VB, Ganesan S, Pazhani GP, Ramamurthy T, Nair GB, Venkatasubramanian P. Storing drinking water in copper pots kills contaminating diarrhoeagenic bacteria. J Health Popul Nutr.

2012 Mar;30(1):17-21. doi: 10.3329/jhpn.v30i1.11271. PMID: 22524115; PMCID: PMC3312355.

Suvorov N, Pogorilaya V, Dyachkova E, Vasil'ev Y, Mironov A, Grin M. Derivatives of Natural Chlorophylls as Agents for Antimicrobial Photodynamic Therapy. Int J Mol Sci. 2021 Jun 15;22(12):6392. doi: 10.3390/ijms22126392. PMID: 34203767; PMCID: PMC8232654.

Stahl, Wilhelm, and Helmut Sies. "β-Carotene and other carotenoids in protection from sunlight." The American Journal of Clinical Nutrition, vol. 96, no. 5, 2012, pp. 1179S-1184S.

Thomson CD, Chisholm A, McLachlan SK, Campbell JM. Brazil nuts: an effective way to improve selenium status. Am J Clin Nutr. 2008 Feb;87(2):379-84. doi: 10.1093/ajcn/87.2.379. PMID: 18258628.

Tello, Carlos, PhD. "25+ Things to Try to Get Rid of Acne (2021)." Health.SelfDecode.Com.

Traber, M. G., & Atkinson, J. (2007). Vitamin E,

Antioxidant and Nothing More. Free Radical Biology and Medicine, 43(1), 4-15. doi: 10.1016/j.freeradbiomed.2007.03.024.

Uwitonze, A. M., & Razzaque, M. S. (2018). Role of Magnesium in Vitamin D Activation and Function. The Journal of the American Osteopathic Association, 118(3), 181–189. doi: 10.7556/jaoa.2018.037.

Varani, J., Warner, R. L., Gharaee-Kermani, M., Phan, S. H., Kang, S., Chung, J. H., ... & Fisher, G. J. (2000). Vitamin A antagonizes decreased cell growth and elevated collagen-degrading matrix metalloproteinases and stimulates collagen accumulation in naturally aged human skin. Journal of Investigative Dermatology, 114(3), 480-486. doi: 10.1046/j.1523-1747.2000.00902.x.

Vaughn, Alexandra R., et al. "Diet and rosacea: the role of dietary change in the management of rosacea." Dermatology Practical & Conceptual, vol. 7, no. 4, 2017, pp. 31–37.

Vaughn AR, Branum A, Sivamani RK. Effects of

Turmeric (Curcuma longa) on Skin Health: A Systematic Review of the Clinical Evidence. Phytother Res. 2016 Aug;30(8):1243-64. doi: 10.1002/ptr.5640. Epub 2016 May 23. PMID: 27213821.

Vostálová J, Tinková E, Biedermann D, Kosina P, Ulrichová J, Rajnochová Svobodová A. Skin Protective Activity of Silymarin and its Flavonolignans. Molecules. 2019 Mar 14;24(6):1022. doi: 10.3390/molecules24061022. PMID: 30875758; PMCID: PMC6470681.

Vollono L, Falconi M, Gaziano R, Iacovelli F, Dika E, Terracciano C, Bianchi L, Campione E. Potential of Curcumin in Skin Disorders. Nutrients. 2019; 11(9):2169. https://doi.org/10.3390/nu11092169

Zakhari, Samir. "Overview: How Is Alcohol Metabolized by the Body?" Alcohol Research & Health, vol. 29, no. 4, 2006, pp. 245–254.

Zaenglein, Andrea L., et al. "Guidelines of care for the management of acne vulgaris." Journal of the American Academy of Dermatology, vol. 74, no. 5, 2016, pp. 945–973.e33.

Zafra-Stone, Sylvia, et al. "Berry anthocyanins as novel antioxidants in human health and disease prevention." Molecular Nutrition & Food Research, vol. 51, no. 6, 2007, pp. 675-683.

BLURB

Dive into "Healthy Skin from Within: The Natural Path to Radiance," your ultimate guide to unlocking your skin's glowing potential through holistic wellness. This book is your personal roadmap to nurturing your body, mind, and spirit, naturally enhancing your inner glow. You'll discover how nutrition, lifestyle, and emotional well-being work together to boost your skin's health and vitality.

Packed with expert insights, practical tips, and personal stories, "Healthy Skin from Within" offers a comprehensive approach to achieving the radiant skin you've always wanted. Perfect for anyone seeking a more authentic and sustainable skincare routine, this book empowers you to make conscious choices that benefit both your skin and the planet.

Whether you're dealing with persistent skin issues or just want to improve your wellness routine, this book is filled with wisdom and inspiration. Start your journey towards a clearer, more vibrant you today. Your adventure to radiant skin awaits!

www.ingramcontent.com/pod-product-compliance
Lightning Source LLC
Chambersburg PA
CBHW051257020426

42333CB00026B/3239